Walking Your Blues Away

"In presenting respectable research and scholarship on how the mundane-seeming, everyday activity of walking balances the brain's laterality, Thom Hartmann brings a scholar's concentration to his subject, a storyteller's sense of enchantment, and a humanitarian's concern with the issues that matter."

STEPHEN LARSEN, AUTHOR OF
THE HEALING POWER OF NEUROFEEDBACK

"Thom Hartmann's work with bilateral movement is a fascinating and important contribution to holistic healing modalities and a timely tool for healing many crises of our modern times."

JAMES ENDREDY, AUTHOR OF
ECOSHAMANISM AND *EARTHWALKS FOR BODY AND SPIRIT*

Walking Your Blues Away

How to Heal the Mind and Create Emotional Well-Being

Thom Hartmann

Park Street Press
Rochester, Vermont

Park Street Press
One Park Street
Rochester, Vermont 05767
www.ParkStPress.com

Park Street Press is a division of Inner Traditions International

Note to the reader: This book is intended as an informational guide. The remedies, approaches, and techniques described herein are meant to supplement, and not to be a substitute for, professional medical care or treatment. They should not be used to treat a serious ailment, including depression and post-traumatic stress disorders, without prior consultation with a qualified health care professional. If you think you have a psychiatric or medical condition, consult a licensed professional.

Library of Congress Cataloging-in-Publication Data

Hartmann, Thom, 1951-
  Walking your blues away : how to heal the mind and create emotional well-being / Thom Hartmann.
     p. cm.
  Includes bibliographical references.
  ISBN-13: 978-1-59477-144-6
  ISBN-10: 1-59477-144-8
  1. Walking—Health aspects. 2. Walking—Psychological aspects. 3. Movement therapy. I. Title.
  RA781.65.H37 2006
  612'.044—dc22

                                                                2006020703

Printed and bound in Canada by Transcontinental Printing

10 9 8 7 6 5 4 3 2 1

Text design and layout by Priscilla Baker
This book was typeset in Sabon, with Eve and Agenda used as display typefaces

To send correspondence to the author of this book, mail a first-class letter to the author c/o Inner Traditions • Bear & Company, One Park Street, Rochester, VT 05767, and we will forward the communication.

To Stan and Cindy Hartmann,
with love and admiration

Contents

Acknowledgments

Special thanks in the preparation of this book go to Susan Davidson, who did an extraordinary job of editing a rough manuscript into a finished book. And to Jeanie Levitan and Jon Graham for bringing it into print. May we all walk a good long way in the journey of life . . .

We Can (and Do!) Heal Ourselves

Healing is a matter of time, but it is sometimes also a matter of opportunity.

HIPPOCRATES

Trauma is nothing new to the human race. We are certainly familiar with trauma in the modern world, from acts of war and terrorism to crime, child abuse, and the pain our dysfunctional, standards-driven schools cause so many of our children. And many of us don't handle trauma well: suicide is the third leading cause of death among Americans ages fifteen to twenty-four.[1] In the last decade over 51 million prescriptions were written in the United States just for the SSRI family of antidepressants (including Prozac, Paxil, and Zoloft), with sales topping $3.6 billion for the six most popular SSRIs, and the numbers have more than doubled since then.[2]

Sociologists may argue about whether early human societies

were comfortable and egalitarian, like many of the modern-day hunter-gatherer peoples living in the world's remaining rain forests, or whether our forebears instead lived in violent dominator cultures ruled by the members who were physically strongest (the fantasy of philosophers and scientists from Rousseau in the seventeenth century to Freud in the twentieth century). However, sociologists and anthropologists and other social thinkers do not disagree that trauma and death have always been part of human life.

So how has humankind historically dealt with trauma for the past two hundred thousand years, before the advent of psychotherapy? Humans experienced mental and emotional wounds in ancient times just as we do today. Family members became sick and died; friends and family were lost to battles with other tribes and with wild animals; after the introduction of agriculture, famine and plagues were periodically visited upon us.

In times past, if four of us set out as a hunting party every few days, odds are that over time at least one person in our party would get eaten by a predator or die in an accident. When that happened right in front of the other three of us, how would we deal with the psychological trauma that resulted from witnessing such an event? We would be in a state of trauma-induced shock. How would we cope with that? How would we deal with the trauma from a near escape from death?

The answer that occurs to most people is that we'd engage in some sort of ritual when we returned to the village, a ritual that usually involved drumming and dancing, two forms of bilateral activity known to induce trance. But this ceremony may have been more to help the people back in the village, such as the family of our lost companion, to work through their grief.

The human body is a self-healing organism. When you cut

your finger, it heals. If you break your leg, it heals. Even if part of you is cut out in surgery, the surgeon's wound heals. We heal from bacterial and viral invasions, from injuries, and from all variety of traumas. The mechanisms for healing are built into us. Five million years of evolution, or the grace of God, or both, have made our bodies automatic healing machines. So why wouldn't the same be true of our minds and emotions?

All of the traumas that we experience in life leave their wounds; if humankind hadn't had ways of healing from those emotional and psychological blows, over time society would have become progressively less functional. Instead, history shows us that people usually recover from even the most severe psychological wounds, often learning great lessons or gaining important insights in the recovery process.

The famous Kauai longitudinal study of children of children raised in stressful, disadvantaged conditions found that a higher percentage of the children grew up "highly resilient" than did a middle-class comparison group.[3] The generation that survived the Great Depression and the Nazi Holocaust in Europe went on to create important social institutions, build nations, and offer comfort and hope to humankind. Elie Wiesel's experience specifically comes to mind: although he would never have wished on another the horrific experience of being in one of Hitler's death camps, through his writing of that experience he has given a particularly inspiring model of resilience and healing to the world.

The reality is that although adversity breaks some people, it strengthens others. And when people heal from adversity, the old cliché of "what doesn't kill you makes you stronger" usually rings true.

But, just as with the production of scar tissue in the healing of a wound to the skin—a process involving millions of cells producing very specific compounds in response to the trauma in the tissue—there must be an inborn mechanism for healing the mind and the emotions. And just as healing from a cut can be speeded up by keeping the wound clean and dry or can be slowed down by letting the wound get wet or dirty or irritated, this emotional healing is also a process that can be either stimulated or thwarted by our interventions.

In this book I've identified a specific healing mechanism and process that nature has built into the human mind and body that enables us to process trauma in a way that is quick, functional, and permanent. Just like the skin's mechanism for forming scabs and scars and eventually even making the scars vanish, this mechanism is simple, fundamental, and elegant.

In its simplest form, this mechanism involves rhythmic side-to-side stimulation of the body. This side-to-side motion, or *bilateral movement,* causes nerve impulses to cross the brain from the left hemisphere to the right hemisphere and back at a specific rate or frequency. This cross-patterning produces an organic integration of left-hemisphere "thinking" functions with right-hemisphere and brain-stem "feeling" functions. This integration is a necessary precursor to emotional and intellectual healing from trauma.

This steady movement of nerve impulses across the hemispheres of the brain is stimulated in the bilateral-movement processes of a variety of modern forms of psychotherapy, such as Eye Movement Desensitization and Reprocessing, Emotional Freedom Technique, and Thought Field Therapy. In its purest form, however, I've discovered that the natural and rhythmic left-right-left-right process of walking, while performing a simple mental exercise, can also stimulate this same internal integration process.

This, I posit, is the way humans have healed themselves from trauma for the hundreds of thousands of years of human history, and it is only because so few of us walk anymore that we have to resort to office-based psychotherapeutic processes to produce the same result.

And that result is impressive. When we stimulate the nervous system in this bilateral manner while calling to mind a persistent emotional distress, the emotional "charge" associated with that memory quickly and permanently dissipates. This isn't a process of producing amnesia or forgetting; instead, it's a way of reframing the past, a way of re-understanding, of putting into context that which has been so "unnerving" for us. When we perform this bilateral process correctly, the pictures of painful past events in our memory transform from stark, scary, sound-filled color movies into black-and-white still pictures that are flattened out and lose their sound. The internal dialogue we have about the events—the "tag line" that we tell ourselves, and actually hear in our own heads in our own voices—changes, usually from something like "That was a painful experience that still scares me" or "I was victimized in that relationship" to a more productive synopsis, such as "Yes, that happened to me, but it's well in the past now and I've learned some good lessons from the experience. I can let go of it."

Inciting the movement of nerve impulses across the brain hemispheres helps people to come to terms with their past. They stop being frightened by their imagined futures and feel comfortable and empowered in the present. Walking while holding a traumatic memory in mind in a particular way can produce this result in a very short time.

This is not new, as you'll discover in this book. Rhythmic bilateral activity as a healing agent has been known to aboriginal peoples for millennia, and in the past few hundred years the secret of using bilaterality to heal emotional and psychological wounds—particularly those that produced psychosomatic physical results—was most famously discovered by Franz Anton Mesmer in the 1700s (called "mesmerism"), refined by Dr. James Braid in the early 1800s (and renamed "hypnosis" by Braid), and brought into widespread and mainstream use in the late 1800s by Sigmund Freud.

However, in an odd historical event in the late 1890s, the growing power of yellow journalism (sensationalized "news" by publishers such as William Randolph Hearst) merged with European anti-Semitism, and the synergy of those forces compelled Freud to abandon these techniques. Freud spent the rest of his life searching in vain for a replacement for hypnosis that actually worked, experimenting with cocaine, developing his early concepts of penis envy and the Oedipal complex, and finally promulgating his largely unsuccessful "talk-therapy" systems. When Freud committed suicide in 1939 he still hadn't found anything that worked as well as the beloved bilateral therapies he'd been forced to abandon by the amazingly synchronous and unusual events of the 1890s.

From the 1890s until the past few decades, hypnosis and the bilateral therapies on which it is based were for the most part ignored or shunned by medical and mental health professionals, in large part because of the uproar of the 1890s. Only with the development of NeuroLinguistic Programming (NLP) in the 1970s, the NLP development of eye-motion therapies, and the 1987 development of Eye Motion Desensitization and Reintegration (EMDR) by Francine Shapiro did bilateral therapies begin to make a comeback.

There is now a whole spectrum of variations on these systems for integrating brain function and thus encouraging healing from psychological and emotional trauma. They all involve stimulating one hemisphere of the brain, then the other, then back to the first, then back again, and repeating this bilateral stimulation over and over. In this book I will show you how you can accomplish this same kind of stimulation using the simple process of walking. This bilateral stimulation gives you access to healing powers, creative states, and emotional and psychological resilience beyond what you may have ever thought possible.

ONE

How Trauma Sticks — The Mechanism of PTSD

*No experience is a cause of success or failure. We do not suf-
fer from the shock of our experience's so-called trauma—but
we make out of them just what suits our purposes.*

ALFRED ADLER

One of the enduring mysteries in the field of psychology is why the
same event produces such different memories and responses in different people. As the *New York Times* reported in a July 1, 2004,
article by Anahad O'Connor, one out of every six soldiers coming
home from the war in Iraq is showing signs of emotional difficul-
ties, particularly post-traumatic stress disorder.

Citing a report in the *New England Journal of Medicine,* the
writer noted, "The researchers surveyed more than 6,000 soldiers

in the months before and after service in Iraq or Afghanistan. Almost 17 percent of those who fought in Iraq reported symptoms of major depression, severe anxiety or post-traumatic stress disorder, compared with about 11 percent of the troops who served in Afghanistan."[1]

In World War II, postwar depression and anxiety was called battle fatigue; in World War I it was referred to as shell shock. The question isn't so much why it happens—we know GIs in war do and see horrific things. The question that perplexes us is why postwar anxiety and depression haunts some veterans and not others. Of course, some vets see harder combat than others. But even that doesn't account for the statistics. There are still huge variations among individual soldiers in how they respond to the same event.

THE LIMBIC BRAIN: THE ONE-DAY SCRATCH PAD

In order to understand why some people are still "shocked" months and even years after a traumatic event, it's necessary to first understand how the brain and the mind process trauma.

The brain is a complex collection of deeply interconnected parts and processes. I will vastly oversimplify here for the purpose of description; this oversimplification is partly for ease of understanding and partly because brain science still doesn't really understand how most of the brain works. (And science certainly doesn't yet understand how memory works.) In light of those caveats, here's a possible scenario that is not inconsistent with much of what is known about brain function and is quite consistent with what we observe "from the outside"—that is, by watching how people react and store information.

9

There is a part of the limbic brain, or visceral brain, called the hippocampus that is believed to function as a one-day scratch pad for memory. Everything you experience throughout the day is stored in the hippocampus; in order for the impressions of the experience to become a long-term memory, they must pass through the hippocampus into the rest of the brain. (People with a damaged hippocampus remember past events but have extreme difficulty learning new things.) Although the rest of the brain is able to integrate recent information from the hippocampus in relation to stored past memories, in order to understand that one thing happened a week ago and another thing happened a month ago, the hippocampus knows only one time: today.

During the night, as we sleep, the hippocampus dumps its information from the day into the rest of the brain for processing, sorting, storing, and disposing of irrelevant information. As the brain is processing the details of the day from the hippocampus, we experience a state that we call "dreaming." Many sleep researchers are convinced that when we experience rapid eye movement (REM) sleep—when our eyes move back and forth rapidly underneath our eyelids—most of the events, including the traumas, of our daily life are processed. The process of information management completed, when we wake up in the morning the hippocampus is once again empty and ready to record another day.

The problem emerges when the hippocampus is carrying information that's too much, or too "hot," for the larger brain/mind to handle. When a recent memory is too strong to be easily and unremarkably processed, it presents in our dream world as a nightmare. If that still doesn't "download" the information from the hippocampus, then the trauma either becomes buried in the subconscious (the process that Freud termed *repression*) or it gets thrown back into the hippocampus the next morning. It's as if the brain says, "Whoa, that's too much for me to process in one evening, so please just hang on to it for now." When the person wakes up the next morning, the information is still there in the hippocampus, still "remembered" and known and felt as if it had happened that very day.

The conjecture that the hippocampus knows little about the more distant past accounts for the unique feature of true post-traumatic stress disorder (PTSD): that the person feels, every day, as if the past event happened today, or in the very recent past. The trauma is always front and center, new, fresh, and raw. The consequences can be psychologically and emotionally disastrous. Every day is affected by a past event: the traumatic event never passes from "now" into "then," and is never processed and filed away in a memory bank, where it loses the power to cause pain and problems on a daily basis. The impact of this on the mind and the emotions is staggering.

Brain scans even demonstrate that before a PTSD event has been processed, the amygdala—a part of the brain responsible for strong emotional states, such as those involved with survival (or the perception of a threat to survival)—and the hippocampus are not functioning normally. The brain scan makes it possible to, in a way, "see" the effect of (or perhaps the mechanism of) the stuck memory. After processing the memory, these parts of the brain usually return to normal functioning.[2]

ACCESS TO RESOURCE STATES

One of the key concepts of many schools of psychology is that human beings are most functional when every part of the mind has access to all other parts. In particular, this functionality is a matter of having full access to positive resources, such as memories of times when we were successful in our undertakings and the good feelings we associate with those accomplishments. Working from this level of functionality, then, when we take on a new task, for example, we first remember times in the past when we attempted something similar and accomplished our goals. This functionality can be accessed in all endeavors, from embarking on a new love relationship to taking on a first public-speaking engagement.

Memories of past accomplishments and capabilities are stored in parts of the brain far from the amygdala and hippocampus. The amygdala and hippocampus, parts of our nervous system's most primary and primitive structures, lie deep in the brain. (Humans share the amygdala and hippocampus structures with all other mammals, unlike our frontal lobes, which we share with only the highest of the apes.) Thus, having a negative memory stuck deep in the hippocampus blocks the pain and fear associated with that memory from reaching and "associating with" positive memories and resource states, which are housed in more-distant parts of the brain.

One of the most elegant and truly useful aspects of walking therapy (and other forms of bilateral intervention) is that, by their very process of side-to-side motion, they cause the right and left lobes of the brain to alternately take responsibility for processing information. Holding your head steady, when you look to your left, the right side of your brain is processing what it is you're seeing. As your line of sight travels past your centerline and to your right, some of the information travels across the corpus callosum, the bundle of nerve fibers that connect the two hemispheres, and is handed off to the left side of the brain for processing.

The two aspects of the hippocampus lie deep within the brain hemispheres, closer to the ancient midbrain than most of the more evolutionarily recent "thinking-function" parts of the brain, which are closer to the surface and generally reside specifically on either the right side or the left side of the brain. This physical/anatomical detail has led researchers to guess that one very significant way in which bilateral therapies function is by keeping the hippocampus (and the amygdala and other parts of the limbic brain and brain stem) engaged through actively recalling the traumatizing memory, while simultaneously and alternately activating the left and right hemispheres of the brain. This process integrates the function of the hippocampus with the two hemispheres of the brain and at the same time connects the two hemispheres. Because the hippocampus is engaged, the processing that would typically happen during sleep happens instead while the person is wide awake, provoking an "emptying" of the hippocampus and the filing and storing of the information it had contained in an appropriate "this-is-the-past" part of the brain.

When people who undergo bilateral therapy wake up the next day, they *know* that what had been bothering them is now in the past. (Often they will dream of the original event overnight.) With the walking therapy that I have developed, in most cases this recognition that the experience is in the past happens during the walk itself. That is the key indicator that the session has been successful.

TWO

Discovering the History of Bilateral Therapies

It still strikes me as strange that the case histories I write
should read like short stories and that, as one might say,
they lack the serious stamp of science.

SIGMUND FREUD, 1895

The first person to develop a system that involved bilateral cross-hemispheric stimulation was a man named Franz Anton Mesmer. In the late 1700s, Mesmer, an Austrian physician who lived in France, healed people of trauma by a variety of techniques that he believed stimulated people's "animal magnetism," which he defined as the animating life force within the human body. To accomplish this healing he sometimes used lodestones (magnets) or water that he had "magnetized." He even claimed to use the direct force of his own "magnetism," including a technique of holding two fingers in front of a patient's face and gently waving the fingers from side to side for a few minutes at a time while the patient held her or his head steady and followed the physician's fingers with the eyes. As Mesmer's biographer James Wyckoff wrote, "Mesmer now considered passes with his hand as the essential part of his cure."[1]

This pioneering physician termed his system mesmerism, and for the latter part of the eighteenth century he was one of the most famous and notorious physicians in Europe. Wolfgang Amadeus Mozart was a friend of Mesmer, and his opera *Bastien et Bastienne* was performed in 1768 in the garden of Mesmer's home. Mozart later wrote Mesmer into his opera *Così fan tutte:*

> *This magnetic stone*
> *Should give the traveler pause.*
> *Once it was used by Mesmer,*
> *Who was born*
> *In Germany's green fields,*
> *And who won great fame*
> *In France.*[2]

Mesmer's system was often highly effective and was widely practiced to treat all manner of physical and psychological ailments, although he was careful not to take patients suffering from clearly "organic" problems such as cancers, sexually transmitted diseases, and other types of obvious infections. Trained as a classical physician, by making this distinction Mesmer was separating out those to whom he either would prescribe medications or would refer to other physicians for surgery or other medical techniques.

Mesmer's special interest was in those conditions caused by a lack of vitality, or *magnetism*—what Freud referred to as hysteria and what today would be considered psychosomatic or psychiatric conditions—those caused by or rooted in emotional trauma. At the height of his career, Mesmer trained hundreds of physicians across Europe in his techniques and had a following that included royalty and people from the highest echelons of society, as well as the most destitute, whom he treated for free.

As happens with many new and unconventional therapies, the medical establishment of his day decided that Mesmer was a threat to them. A "commission of inquiry" was convened, which included a number of France's most well-known physicians, along with the American scientist Benjamin Franklin. The investigators taught themselves what they thought were Mesmer's techniques by having one of his students, d'Eslon, perform mesmerism cures on them. None of them was sick, however, so none was cured.

Recognizing this obvious flaw in their study, the investigators retired to Ben Franklin's home, where, for three days, they tried to repeat what they had seen d'Eslon do, only this time they practiced his techniques on people of "the lower classes."[3] One of the commission members, de Jussieu, got good results and dissented from the majority report, concluding that mesmerism worked. The rest thought it a failure and wrote their opinion in a report dated August 11, 1784. The report, which debunked mesmerism, was a huge blow to Mesmer's reputation and career in France, and caused him to retire to a home in the countryside, where he lived until his death in 1815. He continued to see patients and train doctors, but never again did "grand tours" of the major cities of Europe. Nonetheless, mesmerism and magnetism lived on as healing systems, and were widely practiced all across Europe and the United States well into the nineteenth century.

In November 1841 a French magnetizer by the name of Dr. Charles Lafontaine traveled to England to teach the technique;

in the audience was a Manchester physician of Scottish ancestry named James Braid. Braid was fascinated by the techniques Lafontaine presented, and he began to experiment with them extensively. Braid concluded that Mesmer's claims for the powers of magnets were overstated; the power of trance induction through mesmerism, however, intrigued Braid. He called the phenomenon *neurohypnosis,* later shortening the name of the trance-induction phenomenon to *hypnosis.*

Braid carefully chronicled the aspects of trance states that could be brought about by Mesmer's technique of waving fingers in front of the eyes, so that his patients' eyes moved from side to side while they considered their malady. Braid wrote:

> My first experiments were conceived in view of proving the falseness of the magnetic theory, which states that the provoked phenomena of sleep is the effect of the transmission of the operator on the subject, of some special influence emanating from the first while he makes some touches on the second with the thumb. He looks at him with a fixed stare, while he directs the points of the fingers toward his eyes, and executes some passes in front of him.
>
> It seemed to me that I had clearly established this point, after having taught the subjects to make themselves fall asleep just by fixing an attentive and sustained look on any inanimate object.[4]

To determine whether the technique worked, as Mesmer had believed, because of a magnetic energy moving from the practitioner's fingers to the patient's eyes or whether it instead worked by virtue of the eye motion itself, Braid substituted a swinging pocket watch as the object in motion. The technique still worked, causing

Braid to conclude that the trance states Mesmer induced—and the healing that came from them—were produced more by "fatigue of the eye muscles" or the power of suggestion than by any sort of animal magnetism or etheric field transmitted from practitioner to patient.[5]

Braid and other doctors worked to strip mesmerism of its esoteric content and to arrive at a scientific understanding of the physiological and psychological processes involved in producing trance states by fixed attention and bilateral stimulation through moving the eyes from side to side. At the same time, Andrew Jackson Davis, Madame H. P. Blavatsky, and Phineas Quimby took the esoteric aspects of Mesmer's work and transformed parts of those into the systems that would become Christian Science, Theosophy, and the New Thought movements.

FREUD DISCOVERS HYPNOSIS

The world that Sigmund Freud was born into in 1856 was embracing Braid's refinement of hypnosis with fervor. The practice had spread to hospitals around the world as a means for providing presurgical anesthesia and was being used by many physicians to treat hysteria, a broad category of physical illnesses believed to have a psychological basis. (Those physical illnesses included paralysis, blindness, insomnia, fits, and a wide variety of other conditions.)

When Freud was twenty-four years old and just out of medical school, his mentor, Josef Breuer, began treating a twenty-one-year-old Orthodox Jewish woman named Bertha Pappenheim, whom Freud referred to in writing as Anna O. The young woman had spent several years of her life nursing her ailing father; when he died she developed a number of illnesses, including periodic mute-ness, paralysis, hallucinations, and spasms. Though she lived in Germany, she refused to speak German; she would converse only in English. She had tried on several occasions to kill herself.

At the time, therapeutic hypnotic methods varied to some degree, although most involved the classic technique of having a patient fix her or his attention on one point. In a paper published in 1881, Freud wrote of several hypnosis techniques he and Breuer preferred. One was clearly handed down from Mesmer: Freud wrote that "we sit down opposite the patient and request him to fixate on two fingers on the physician's right hand and at the same time to observe closely the sensations which develop."[6]

The other technique seemed a more recent invention of Breuer's and Freud's and involved, as Freud wrote, "stroking the patient's face and body with both hands continuously for from five to ten minutes," a technique quite useful for calming "hysterical" female patients. Freud noted that "this has a strikingly soothing and lulling effect." The "stroking" that Freud and Breuer practiced involved alternately stroking the left, then the right side of the body, a technique Mesmer had first developed.[7]

Breuer treated Bertha with these and other hypnotic techniques to some success, although Freud observed that in the process the woman fell in love with Breuer, a married man old enough to be her father. Bertha claimed Breuer had impregnated her and that she would have his baby; Breuer claimed she had a "hysterical pregnancy." She was moved to a private sanitarium, where she lived for the next few years out of the public eye. To this day it is not known whether the pregnancy was terminated by abortion or miscarriage, whether she gave birth, or whether, as Breuer claimed, her pregnancy symptoms were all the result of her "hysterical" desire to have his child and had no basis in physical reality.

What is known is that, after her release from the sanitarium, Bertha Pappenheim never again discussed Breuer or Freud, but instead became Germany's first and most outspoken social worker and feminist. She rose to Susan B. Anthony–like fame in Germany, writing books and producing plays advocating women's rights, and translating into German and publishing Mary Wollstonecraft's 1792 groundbreaking treatise on women's rights, *A Vindication of the Rights of Women*. In 1904 she founded a Jewish women's movement, the Jüdischer Frauenbund, which was so influential in Germany that it came to the attention of the Nazis; she died after being interrogated by Hitler's thugs in 1936. She had never married or, as far as can be ascertained, ever had a relationship with a man after her claim of impregnation by Breuer.

In the first year of her treatment by Breuer, Bertha had found that it was very useful for her to spend long hours talking with the attentive Breuer about her feelings: she called this her "talk therapy" and "chimney sweeping." He would come to her home both evenings and mornings to hear her "talk therapy." Even though Freud and Breuer never claimed this talk therapy to be a "cure," her case became the cornerstone of Freud's theories and of modern talk-based psychotherapies.

But in the 1880s and early 1890s, talk therapy wasn't Freud's favorite or even most common form of treatment for his patients. At the time, Freud's treatment methodology of choice was a bilateral eye-motion technique known as hypnosis.

In his 1893 *Some Points for a Comparative Study of Organic and Hysterical Motor Paralyses* and his 1895 *Studies on Hysteria* (the "founding document" on Freudian psychoanalysis, which was coauthored with Josef Breuer), Freud based nearly all of his conclusions on results he obtained using Mesmer's and Braid's eye-motion and other hypnotic techniques. In *Studies on Hysteria,* for example, Freud wrote: "Quite frequently it is some event in child-hood that sets up a more or less severe symptom which persists during the years that follow. Not until they have been questioned *under hypnosis* [my italics] do these memories emerge with the undiminished vividness of a recent event."[8]

In 1893 Freud published *On the Psychical Mechanism of Hysterical Phenomena: Preliminary Communication,* coauthored with Josef Breuer. In it he addressed the subject of hypnosis frequently and explicitly. "As a rule, it is necessary to hypnotize the patient and to arouse memories under hypnosis," he wrote in the opening paragraph of the paper. "When this [hypnosis] is done, it becomes possible to demonstrate the connection in the clearest and most convincing fashion." As always, his technique involved using his hand or a watch to move the patient's eyes from side to side, and occasionally stroking the patient on alternate sides of her body.[9]

In the paper, Freud and Breuer refer to their learning hypnotic techniques in 1881, and refer to their work before 1881 as "the 'pre-suggestion' era."[10] Repeatedly, Freud and Breuer referred to the power of hypnosis for both diagnostic and therapeutic work. They suggested that the root causes of hysteria are found in old memories or emotional traumas, and that "Not until [the patients] have been questioned under hypnosis do these memories emerge."[11]

And the cure for these painful old memories that are driving neurotic behavior? Freud and Breuer wrote: "It will now be understood how it is that the psychotherapeutic procedure which we have described in these pages has a curative effect. *It brings to an end the operative force of the idea which was not abreacted in the first instance, by allowing its strangulated affect to find a way out through speech; and it subjects it to associative correction by introducing it into normal consciousness under light hypnosis or by removing it through the physician's suggestion, as is done in somnambulism* [hypnosis] *accompanied by amnesia."*[12]

Freud's main technique for inducing what he called somnambulism was to wave his hand or his fingers from side to side in front of his patient's face while suggesting that the person relax and then consider her or his problem or issue. Freud also used techniques borrowed from stage hypnotists, including "tapping," a technique wherein Freud alternately tapped two fingertips on the person's forehead, cheeks, or collarbone, continually from left to right, until a trance was induced, and another technique in which he put his hand on the client's forehead and applied increasing pressure.

Hypnotic-induction techniques such as these were used to treat people across Europe and America; Freud was using quick-induction trance states to give him access to the inner workings of his patients' minds, helping him to flesh out his theory of the unconscious.

But hypnosis was not uncontroversial. Ever since the father of one of Mesmer's young female patients forced his way into Mesmer's treatment room to "rescue" his daughter, the misuse of hypnosis was a hot topic. Stage demonstrations of hypnosis were among the most popular forms of entertainment throughout the mid- and late 1800s, and usually involved a beautiful female assistant who was put into a trance and then commanded to give blind obedience to the hypnotist.

In 1885, the novelist Jules Clarette published in Paris a work of fiction titled *Jean Mornas,* about a hypnotist who caused people to steal for him and left them with no memory of the events. In July 1886, as the novel was being translated into German and English, the French *Revue De l'Hypnotisme* magazine published the results of a series of experiments that sensationalized Clarette's novel: in those experiments, physicians hypnotized their patients and then successfully commanded them to steal. The revelations of these experiments were very troubling to the French public. When *Jean Mornas* appeared in German in 1889, its publication caused quite a sensation.

By 1891, Freud was still writing enthusiastically about hypnosis, claiming that he had "become convinced that quite a number of symptoms of organic diseases are accessible to hypnosis," but, backpedaling because of the bad press surrounding Clarette's novel, Freud added that "in view of the dislike of hypnotic treatment prevailing at present, it seldom comes about that we can employ hypnosis except after all other kinds of treatment have been tried without success."[13]

Nonetheless, Freud continued to use hypnosis—particularly bilateral eye-motion induction techniques—and continued to get good results from the technique. And he wasn't alone in this: by 1890 most psychiatrists were using the finger-waving-before-the-eyes "hypnotism" system to produce rapid psychotherapeutic results. Braid's refinement of Mesmer's technique was used almost universally across the psychiatry community, and all indications are that it was producing positive results for many patients.

In 1894, however, George Du Maurier changed all that.

FREUD'S CHANGE OF COURSE

Most people alive today won't remember Du Maurier's name, or even the title of his notorious work of fiction; most people do, however, recognize the name of the villain Du Maurier created. Du Maurier's novel *Trilby*, published in 1894, became a worldwide best seller in its day and still stands as one of the most famous books of the nineteenth century.

Trilby played on both the growing public fear of hypnosis and the new wave of anti-Semitism that was building in Europe at the end of the nineteenth century. Du Maurier described his villain in explicit and stereotypical terms:

> First, a tall bony individual of any age between thirty and forty-five, of Jewish aspect, well-featured but sinister. He was very shabby and dirty, and wore a red béret and a large velveteen cloak, with a big metal clasp at the collar. His thick, heavy, languid, lusterless black hair fell down behind his ears on to his shoulders, in that musician-like way that is so offensive to the normal Englishman. He had bold, brilliant black eyes, with long heavy lids, a thin, sallow face, and a beard of burnt-up black which grew almost from his under eyelids; and over it his mustache, a shade lighter, fell in two long spiral twists. He went by the name of Svengali, and spoke fluent French with a German accent, and humorous German twists and idioms, and his voice was very thick and mean and harsh, and often broke into a disagreeable falsetto.[14]

Du Maurier's villain, Svengali, was an unemployed musician who used hypnosis to put a beautiful young woman named Trilby under his spell. Svengali brought Trilby into a trance using the same methods Freud was using with his clients and that many stage hypnotists were then using as well: bilateral eye movement and tapping her forehead, cheeks, and upper chest left–right, left–right.

Du Maurier wrote:

> Svengali told her to sit down on the divan, and sat opposite to her, and bade her look him well in the white of the eyes. "Recartez-moi pien tans le blanc tes yeaux" [Look into the whites of my eyes]. Then he made little passes and counterpasses on her forehead and temples and down her cheek and neck. Soon her eyes closed and her face grew placid.[15]

Once Trilby was under Svengali's power, he mercilessly exploited her sexually and financially until, at the end of the story, she dies tragically of exhaustion while staring at Svengali's picture.

The publication of *Trilby* was accompanied by several incidents that made headlines in Europe and America during 1894 and 1895. Stage hypnotist Ceslav Lubicz-Czynski allegedly used hypnosis to seduce the baroness Hedwig von Zedlitz, which caused her family to report him to the police. According to the (increasingly hysterical) press, another stage hypnotist, Franz Neukomm, suggested to his subject that she "leave her body" for astral travel to heal another person on the stage. Newspaper stories said the woman died because of that suggestion, leading to headlines that fairly screamed "Hypnosis Voodoo Death!"

Even Alexander Dumas, the author of *The Three Musketeers,* wrote several novels during this era that employed hypnosis and its power to seduce and control others—particularly women—as a major plot device.

The lurid stories spread worldwide, bringing hypnosis and the bilateral-induction techniques associated with it into disrepute. No matter how effective the technique of having patients concentrate while either moving their eyes from side to side or being tapped on either side of the face, it was not to be done any more.

No physician—and particularly no Jewish physician—would in his right mind be willing to take the risk of being accused of using what the newspapers had decided was Svengali's "evil power" of hypnosis, even if hypnosis did have the power to heal. And Breuer and Freud were both Jewish physicians.

Freud's frustration with having to abandon his eye-motion and hypnotic therapies must have been extreme, but public reaction to the 1894 publication of *Trilby* and the lurid hypnosis stories that accompanied it were so intense that I postulate he had no other choice. With the simple technique of generating healing through moving his fingers in front of patients' eyes denied him by public opinion, Freud abandoned hypnosis in 1895 and turned to drugs as a way of treating neuroses.

From 1895 to 1897, Freud gave cocaine to virtually all of his patients, himself also regularly ingesting small doses of the drug. As he wrote in *On Cocaine:*

A few minutes after taking cocaine, one experiences a certain exhilaration and feeling of lightness. One feels a certain furriness on the lips and palate, followed by a feeling of warmth in the same areas; if one now drinks cold water, it feels warm on the lips and cold in the throat. . . . During this first trial I experienced a short period of toxic effects, which did not recur in subsequent experiments. Breathing became slower and deeper and I felt tired and sleepy; I yawned frequently and felt somewhat dull. After a few minutes the actual cocaine euphoria began, introduced by repeated cooling eructation. Immediately after taking the cocaine I noticed a slight slackening of the pulse and later a moderate increase. . . . On the whole the toxic effects of coca are of short duration, and much less intense than those produced by effective doses of quinine or salicylate of soda; they seem to become even weaker after repeated use of cocaine.[16]

Interestingly, to this day most students of Freud have not connected the international furor over hypnosis that was ignited in 1895 by *Trilby* with the timeline of Freud's life and explorations. For instance, in an article titled "Sigmund Freud und Cocaine" published in the German-language *Wien Klin Wochenschr,* author G. Lebzeltern muses: "The basic tenet proposed by J. V. Scheidt states that the narcotic drug cocaine played a role in the development of psychoanalysis, which has been underestimated up to the present day. It is a fact that Freud himself took cocaine (in small doses) for about two years, and that he began his dream interpretation approximately ten years later. . . . The question to be answered now is: Why did this happen [begin] precisely in 1895?"[17]

The article then goes on to suggest personal psychological reasons for why Freud started using cocaine as therapy in 1895, stopped using cocaine in 1897, in the fall of that year proposed the Oedipus complex as the basis for much neurosis, and then turned to dream therapy ten years later. However, if you superimpose the historical timelines of the development of hypnosis as therapy and as stagecraft and the publication of *Jean Mornas* and of *Trilby* on the timeline of Freud's life and work, the simple fact emerges that Freud stopped practicing Mesmer's technique of rhythmically moving his fingers in front of his patients' eyes or repeatedly tapping alternate sides of the face and upper chest at the same time that the newspapers had branded that practice as "black magic" and had determined that it was a ploy used by Jewish men to seduce and exploit vulnerable women.

At that time, all doctors were men and nearly all of the psychiatric patients were women. In the wake of the *Trilby*-induced hysteria of 1895, in all probability Freud couldn't have continued using Mesmer's version of eye-motion therapy even if he wanted to: virtually all of his patients were women from the educated classes who read newspapers and novels, and would likely have run from the office screaming if their physician tried using the same well-publicized methods the fictional Svengali employed to seduce and exploit the unfortunate Trilby.

Nonetheless, Freud continued to hold his conviction of the power of having his clients move their eyes from side to side, or tapping on alternate sides of the body—what at that time he referred to as "hypnosis." But it took him almost thirty years to again even mention hypnosis in public. In 1923, in *Psychoanalysis: Exploring the Hidden Recesses of the Mind,* Freud wrote: "The importance of hypnotism for the history of the development of psychoanalysis must not be too lightly estimated. Both in theoretic as well as in therapeutic aspects, psychoanalysis is the administrator of the estate left by hypnotism."[18]

But, convictions aside, the year 1895 was to mark the end of Freud's use of hypnosis. Right up to the day he committed suicide with a morphine overdose on September 23, 1939, he never again publicly used or advocated the techniques employed by Mesmer, Braid, and the fictional Svengali.

Freud's body of work that emerged post-1895 has not well withstood the test of time. Although Freudian analysis is still practiced around the world, there are no clean scientific studies that support the efficacy of Freudian psychotherapy or many of the offshoots it has spawned. Drawing on the case of Bertha Pappenheim, Freud concluded that her "talk-therapy" sessions every morning and evening with Josef Breuer, which included many emotional outbursts as she told of her earlier experiences, were a cathartic abreaction process similar to lancing a boil. Although Freud and Breuer freely acknowledge that Bertha wasn't "cured" by this talk-therapy process, Freud nonetheless built an entire therapeutic model on it. (Breuer went back into family medicine after his one experience in psychiatry with Bertha.)

Many observers of the psychology/psychiatry scene have noted over the years how ironic it is that Freud's psychotherapeutic legacy was founded on a single case that ended with his patient having to be involuntarily hospitalized. Yet he and his disciples became famous largely because of his other (unpublished) early successes. In the years prior to 1895, Freud relied almost entirely on bilateral techniques, and had profound and lasting successes, the stories of which traveled by word of mouth through the psychiatric community and the upper echelons of society, bringing him patients from around the world.

Many historians of psychotherapy have speculated over the past century about why Freud abandoned his early successful quick-therapy bilateral techniques for his later techniques that required years of commitment and were for the most part unsuccessful. The most cynical have suggested that Freud was simply building a practice and an industry that would sustain itself financially because patients would have to come back regularly over a period of years, providing a good income for the therapist.

The truth is probably more flattering to Freud: He had to stop using hypnosis because of a fiction-inspired hysteria that swept the world so powerfully that he couldn't defend himself against it, even though truth was on his side.

Because Freud's "secret" lay hidden for almost a century, millions of people the world over were denied the benefits of the rapid-healing techniques he called hypnotism, a process grounded in the simple practice of alternately stimulating the two hemispheres of the brain while thinking of a problem or issue. Society as a whole was also denied a discussion of bilaterality and its broader implications for cultural development.

THREE

Why Bilaterality Is So Important

Never trust a thought that didn't come by walking.

FRIEDRICH NIETZSCHE

Bilaterality is the ability to have the left and the right hemispheres of the brain fully functional and communicating with each other. It represents an optimal way of functioning for the brain, a way that reflects how most animals' brains operate.

Many people in our society are "stuck" in a groove of habitual emotional response, with only one hemisphere of the brain taking responsibility for much of the brain's functioning. Even though they're "normal" and "sane," they're carrying around a mind full of unresolved emotion and pain. Bilateral exercises have been demonstrated to encourage healthier brain functionality. Now we're finding that walking can also perform this healing.

As recently as thirty years ago, before the availability of

sophisticated brain-imaging equipment such as PET, SPECT, and MRI scanners, it was widely believed that the left hemisphere of the brain—which controls the right side of the body—was responsible for logic and thinking, and the right hemisphere—which controls the left side of the body—took charge of emotions. Interestingly, though we now know that it's not quite that simple, we also know that there is a significant grain of truth in this long-standing belief.

A healthy person operates with both hemispheres of the brain fully engaged and able to hand off information to one another in such a way that we can think about our emotions and evoke feelings with our thoughts. Evidence of this dual-hemispheric functioning can be recognized by simply watching an able-bodied person walk or talk—both sides of the mouth open the same amount when the person speaks, and both legs and arms swing comfortably and reach the same distances when they walk. A person who is said to "speak out of one side of his mouth" is showing signs either of single hemispheric brain damage (such as from a stroke) or of serious emotional or psychological illness. One hemisphere has taken over the brain's functioning. Depending on which hemisphere has taken charge, such people often either are overly emotional (usually left-side-of-the-mouth speakers) or are lacking the ability to easily experience emotions (right-side speakers). Our culture has intuited this for hundreds of years—thus the old expression about a person "speaking out of one side of his mouth."

Hemispheric dominance—one side of the brain controlling the functions of both—is no small matter, and not only has an effect on individuals but, some scientists suggest, actually shapes society and culture itself. In a very real way, even though most of us talk out of both sides of the mouth, a *cultural* hemispheric dominance is reflected in societies that we call "civilized," whereas indige-nous/aboriginal societies (Rousseau's "noble savages") are more bilateral in their overall cultural brain functioning.

Just as a person with a severe hemispheric imbalance can be badly disconnected from emotions such as empathy, and thus sanc-tion or even encourage actions such as the mass murder that is war, so too can an entire society. In the opinion of some research-ers, societies that are hemispherically unbalanced are more likely to be patriarchial, hierarchical, and violent, whereas societies that are hemispherically balanced are more likely to be egalitarian and democratic, and employ violence only in self-defense.

What we now call *civilization*—the earliest example of an entire culture becoming left-hemisphere dominant—can be traced back to the oldest written tale, *The Epic of Gilgamesh,* a story set six to seven thousand years ago in ancient Mesopotamia (now Iraq) about the first ruler to defy the gods and seize control of others in the process. Gilgamesh was history's first warlord. His epic tale, which predates the Bible, describes not only a hierarchical social order but a hierarchical religion as well: it tells the story of a good man named Utnapishtim who was told by his god, Ea, to build an ark and put into it two of every animal. By doing this, Utnapishtim survives a great flood that Ea brings upon the city of Shurippak because its people aren't sufficiently worshipful of Ea.

Gilgamesh's culture established, in many ways, the prototype for later agriculture-based (and violence-based) social and political systems. A regnant king or queen with the power to remove the head of any person who dared defy him or her ruled every civili-zation from Gilgamesh's Mesopotamia to today's Saudi Arabia. Whether east or west, north or south, from China to Europe to the Inca, violent dominator societies have emerged over the past few thousand years. With millennia of this history as background, by the turn of the nineteenth century Darwin and others of his era reasoned that Gilgamesh's dominance-based model must be the way humans were *meant* to live.

In his 1871 book, *The Descent of Man,* Charles Darwin summarized the notion, common at the time, that society is best held together by dominance rather than true democracy, by the elite few rather than the unwashed masses, by those most willing to wield force rather than those willing to compromise or sacrifice. Darwin was making the case that most humans are biologically predisposed to living under the dominance of others.

The assumption of conquerors has always been that they are superior in every way to the conquered. How else does one justify the conquest?

Darwin, however, had a problem making his view fit into what he was learning about the social models of the tribal peoples he and his contemporaries called savages. Reports were beginning to trickle in to the scientific and political communities from explorers and colonists in the New World and the African and Indian colonies that these so-called savages—tribal peoples from the Americas to Africa—weren't the stupid, selfish, and violent characters they'd been portrayed as in European literature and philosophy. Instead, they often displayed altruistic behavior and had social and political systems that were highly sophisticated, and in many cases were far more democratic than was England in Darwin's day.

At the time there were about as many indigenous peoples living tribally around the world as there were "civilized" people. They were living the way all humans had lived for most of human history (and thus were often referred to as "Stone Age people"), and yet their societies were troublingly democratic. Pesky Americans such as Thomas Jefferson and Benjamin Franklin had written and spoken extensively about the lessons to be learned from the democratic forms of governance of the savages of North America. And the savages of Asia and Africa often lived peacefully, cooperatively, and with elaborate and sophisticated—but egalitarian—social organizations as well. Even though two centuries earlier Thomas Hobbes had proclaimed "Life in an unregulated state of nature is solitary, poor, nasty, brutish, and short," there was little evidence to be found of such living conditions among the "unregulated" tribal peoples of the time.

Presumably Darwin's ancestors had once been savages, too. Why, Darwin wondered, hadn't the modern-day savages being found in the Americas and elsewhere developed into "civilized" societies, as Darwin's fellow Englishmen had?

"It is, however, very difficult to form any judgment," Darwin wrote, "[as to] why one particular tribe and not another has been successful and has risen in the scale of civilisation. Many savages are in the same condition as when first discovered several centuries ago. As Mr. Bagehot [the economist and political writer Walter Bagehot] has remarked, we are apt to look at progress as normal in human society; but history refutes this."

Why did modern tribal peoples of the time live the way they did, even when offered an opportunity to become "civilized"? The stories of Native Americans brought up in white communities who later escaped back into the "savage wilds" were legendary; similarly, Africans fiercely resisted being taken into white communities as slaves, even though it represented a "civilized" improvement over their tribal conditions. As well, it was not uncommon during colonial days for Europeans to escape to Indian communities to live among them, becoming "white Indians" and never returning to "civilized" society. This intrigued Thomas Jefferson, who began a detailed analysis of Native American peoples and societies. As Jefferson wrote in his autobiographical *Notes on Virginia:*

> Founded on what I have seen of man, white, red, and black, and what has been written of him by authors, enlightened themselves, and writing among an enlightened people, the Indian of North America being more within our reach, I can speak of him somewhat from my own knowledge, but more from the information of others better acquainted with him, and on whose truth and judgment I can rely. . . . [H]e is brave, when an enterprise depends on bravery; education with him making the point of honor consist in the destruction of an enemy by stratagem, and in the preservation of his own person free from injury; . . . also, he meets death with more deliberation, and endures tortures with a firmness unknown almost to religious enthusiasm with us; that he is affectionate to his children, careful of them, and indulgent in the extreme; that his affections comprehend his other connections; weakening, as with us, from circle to circle, as they recede from the centre; that his friendships are strong and faithful to the uttermost extremity, that his sensibility is keen, even the warriors weeping most bitterly on the loss of their children, though in general they endeavor to appear superior to human events; that his vivacity and activity of mind is equal to ours in the same situation; hence his eagerness for hunting, and for games of chance. . . .
>
> They raise fewer children than we do. . . . It is said, therefore, that they have learned the practice of procuring abortion by the

use of some vegetable; and that it even extends to prevent conception for a considerable time after. . . . An inhuman practice once prevailed in this country, of making slaves of the Indians. . . . To judge of the truth of this, to form a just estimate of their genius and mental powers, more facts are wanting, and great allowance to be made for those circumstances of their situation which call for a display of particular talents only. This done, we shall probably find that they are formed in mind as well as in body, on the same module with the "Homo sapiens Europaeus."[1]

As suggested by Jefferson's description of Native peoples and their character and customs, there had to be something Darwin was missing in the theory of why "savages" didn't want to become "civilized," but Darwin couldn't figure out what it was. A theory suggesting that "savages" had actually begun as "civilized people" but had deteriorated or degenerated over the eons was put forth by the duke of Argyll, although Darwin found that wanting. "The arguments recently advanced by the Duke of Argyll and formerly by Archbishop Whately, in favour of the belief that man came into the world as a civilised being, and that all savages have since undergone degradation, seem to me weak in comparison with those advanced on the other side," Darwin wrote in *The Descent of Man*.[2] And yet he had no way to account for the apparent nobility and quality of life among the savages.

Darwin was a scientist, and he knew that meant sometimes bringing forward unpopular views. Flipping Argyll's theory upside down, Darwin began to consider that perhaps civilized people had once been savages, too. But if civilized people *had* once lived as savages, why didn't we remember those times?

THE CULTURAL DISSOCIATIVE BARRIER

In his brilliant *Ishmael* books, Daniel Quinn popularizes the idea of a memory barrier between modern civilization and what Darwin called the "savage" state.[3] Quinn calls this "The Great Forgetting," a cultural amnesia so strong that we're unable even to *imagine* how our ancestors lived.

For example, when we think of another "civilized" country, we imagine our stereotypes of people in full color: Greeks dancing like Zorba, or French women and men sipping wine, or Italians eating pasta in a café in Venice. Even if we don't speak their language, we can hear fragments of it, and can easily imagine them speaking the language. We can bring to mind the smells, tastes, and even the feel of their world, because on the whole it is so culturally similar to our own.

But when we think of our own ancestors' preliterate history, our mindscape often turns to black-and-white. Our ability to imagine language or other sounds from that time is minimal. (Indeed, up to the past decade, some anthropologists speculated that our "savage" ancestors were mute, suggesting that the development of civilization coincided with a recent evolutionary mutation that increased the size of the nerve bundles that control the human tongue.) Most people have never tried to conjure up a sense of what the food of our prehistoric ancestors must have tasted like; what sorts of herbs, seeds, and pollens they used as spices; how their living areas smelled; or what brought them joy.

We all have a collection of different "selves," or roles, that we necessarily play in life: parent, teacher, employee, spouse, friend. Each role requires us to move slightly different skill sets and personality attributes front and center when engaging one of these selves. When a person loses the ability to remember that he or she carries the same identity when acting out various roles, that person is said to have developed a dissociative disorder. Multiple-personality disorder is the most well known of these.

Collectively, it appears that we've erected a cultural dissociative barrier that is so complete that we believe Darwin was right in his assumption that a dominance- and violence-based culture is biologically based, and has grown and thrived because of natural selection.

THE LEFT BRAIN TAKES OVER

Into this centuries-old debate about why "civilized" society is so violent and "savages" are often so nonviolent steps modern brain science. In 1982, Walter J. Ong published a book titled *Orality and Literacy,* in which he suggests that there was a profound difference in the way brains developed in cultures that learned to read at an early age versus cultures that were entirely oral in the way they passed along stories, mores, and social traditions.[4] In 1999, physician and science writer Leonard Shlain expanded on this hypothesis in his book *The Alphabet Versus the Goddess: The Conflict Between Word and Image,* suggesting that the process of learning to read is an entirely left-brain exercise that causes children to develop left-hemisphere brain dominance at an early age.[5]

The left hemisphere (which controls the right side of the body) is largely responsible for abstract and logical thought. Alphabets are pure abstractions—there is nothing about the shape or characters of the word *bird,* for instance, that would cause somebody who didn't read to know that this particular collection of symbols refers to a feathered creature. Thus, learning to read is a process that works out the left brain, and exercising this side of the brain prior to the age of seven—roughly the age when hemispheric dominance is determined—will cause people to develop left-hemisphere dominance rather than the more functional right-brain/left-brain bilaterality.

As more and more people in a society become literate, and therefore left-brain dominant, Shlain suggests, they also become more disconnected from their emotional and empathic right-brain side. Shlain suggests that this early left-hemispheric dominance and disconnection from the empathic right-brain self means that we become more willing (or even driven) to use violence, particularly men against women. He presents evidence of this by showing how time waves of literacy in Europe have corresponded with alternating waves of goddess worship (in the form of Mary cults during times when it was illegal to read), noting that, within a generation of the widespread introduction of literacy to Europe, the Catholic Church and its Inquisition murdered over a million women as "witches" as part of their determined effort to stamp out the cults that worshipped the divinity of Mary. With left-hemispheric dominance spreading across the culture, the men rose up and took over in a brutal and bloody way.

Thus, Shlain, Ong, and others suggest that *literacy* is the element in the soup pot of civilization that irrevocably altered the way "civilized society" developed. Because literacy changes how our brains are forming as we grow and develop, we have no reference point for understanding how we may have been had we not grown up literate, and thus no ability to truly understand or empathize with nonliterate and nonviolent societies. The result is that we assume that nonviolent societies can't really exist, and that our type of brain development is "normal" for the human race.

Whether bilateral walking therapy in and of itself is enough to cure many of the violent ills of society is doubtful, but conceivable. The Indians of North America were pedestrians before the introduction of the horse from Europe in the 1500s, and available anthropologic evidence indicates that their societies were rarely violent.[6] With the widespread use of non-walking forms of transportation in Europe and the Middle East seven thousand years ago (primarily the horse and the horse-drawn carriage and chariot), it's possible the loss of walking made society more violent.

Even glimpses we get today of societies that still depend entirely on walking for transportation—such as the San of southern Africa, who were featured in the movie *The Gods Must Be Crazy*—find that "walking" people are rarely as violent or as hierarchical as "riding" people.

Although all of it is speculative at this moment, the evidence is accumulating that both social and personal mental health depend on people having regular bilateral stimulation, and that we're evolutionarily designed to derive that from daily walking.

——⚬⚬⚬——

FOUR

NLP and the Modern History of Bilateral Therapies

O imitators, you slavish herd!

HORACE, 65 BCE–8 BCE

For just over sixty years—from the turn of the last century, when Freud abandoned the practice of moving his fingers back and forth in front of his patients' faces, until the 1950s, when Milton Erickson and others began to gain acceptance for their efforts to revive the practice of therapeutic hypnosis—the only way a person could use eye-motion therapy to heal from trauma was during rapid eye movement (REM) sleep. While REM sleep is important and useful, and—as we discussed in the first chapter—is apparently one way in which the normal vicissitudes of life are processed, REM sleep often isn't strong enough to process severe trauma.

The human potential movement that began to flourish in the late 1960s provided fertile ground for developing new perspectives on how the human mind works. In the early 1970s, John Grinder, an assistant professor of linguistics at the University of California at Santa Cruz, and Richard Bandler, a fourth-year undergraduate involved in Gestalt therapy, teamed up to develop a model for how the mind and body interact. Under the mentorship of Gregory Bateson, the two created the model and system known as NeuroLinguistic Programming, defining a relationship between the mind *(neuro)* and language, both verbal and nonverbal *(linguistic)*, and suggesting how their interaction might be organized *(programming)* to affect mind, body, and behavior.[1]

Eye Motion Therapy (EMT) came out of the early work of Richard Bandler and John Grinder. In the process of developing NLP, the founders noticed that each emotional state and each memory a person carried has its own unique sensory structure. A memory will exist in color or in black-and-white, as a still picture or as a movie, and it will have a sound element or it won't. If you ask a person to point to the memory, that person will point in a particular direction and will be able to tell you if he or she experiences the picture of the memory as being two feet away or twenty feet away. Generally, recent and/or emotionally intense memories are closer and more likely to be color filled, and often are seen as if the person was an observer (that is, he doesn't see himself in the picture), whereas older and less emotion-charged images are more distant and faded or lacking color, and often the person can see himself in the picture.

Grinder and Bandler observed that people tend to internalize unprocessed and unresolved memories of traumatic events in bright, full color; the memory sounds are usually loud and the memory feelings intense. They discovered that when people shifted these structural components of the traumatic memory—the specific visual, auditory, and kinesthetic qualities (which they called *submodalities*) of their internal mental pictures and memories of events—the emotional charge of those events shifted. They deduced that the structural components of memory are part of the mind's way of organizing and giving meaning to memories—the mind's "filing and organizing system"—*and* are the key to therapeutically changing them.

For example, you might remember a time of embarrassment as a bright color picture on your left side, about five feet away from you. If you move that picture to the upper right corner of your field of vision, push it twenty feet out, and then turn from color to black-and-white, the odds are high that the emotional charge associated with the memory will diminish. Bandler and Grinder call this process *shifting the submodalities.*

One of the most important submodalities of a memory, Bandler and Grinder found, is position. Thus, early NLP practitioners such as Bandler and Steve Andreas had people move their memory pictures back and forth and back and forth to see what would happen. The result was that with *minor* emotional traumas, this lateral movement of the pictures rapidly "flattened" the picture, reducing the emotional charge.

This discovery about moving pictures from side to side, Richard Bandler told me, was a fascinating insight into the power of bilateral stimulation and functions. "If you're just tossing a tennis ball from hand to hand," he said, "it's impossible to feel angry, and if you do it while thinking of a problem, often the problem will resolve or solutions will pop into your mind."

There was only one problem with the initial system of having people move their traumatic memory pictures from side to side. For *big* traumas, this "brute force" method would sometimes bring back to people the intensity of the event so strongly and quickly that they'd break into tears or "freak out"—an experience known as an *abreaction*. Although Sigmund Freud had considered abreactions generally a good thing and thought it a sign of healing when patients broke down and cried or went into distress during their therapy sessions with him, experience had taught Bandler and Grinder that this was actually a re-wounding that left people in greater emotional distress than before they experienced the abreaction. (Numerous studies in the past five decades have proved this to be true. Many abreaction-based therapies that were popular in the 1960s, such as screaming and hitting pillows with baseball bats, have been discredited and discontinued because evoking abreactions to relive a trauma can be so emotionally harmful.)

This desire to avoid abreactions led to a search for ways to create true structural change in memories without producing a re-wounding response. To avoid abreactions, then, they suggested a person hold the memory picture in one place; while the person held the memory picture in place—say, a few feet in front of the chest, which seems to be where most people hold highly traumatic pictures—they'd have the person move his or her eyes from side to side, following the tip of a pen held in the hand of the NLP practitioner.

NeuroLinguistic Programming researchers discovered that if the tip of the pen the person was following with his or her eyes didn't "touch" the picture, there was no abreaction and the intensity of the picture would gradually diminish. When the NLP practitioner did this several times for a few minutes each time, until the pen tip had moved back and forth over the top of the picture enough to reduce the emotional intensity of the picture by at least 50 percent, then the person would not experience an abreaction when the practitioner finally *did* move the pen (and thus the person's vision) into the area that the memory picture occupied. When the pen finally "punctured" the picture, the resolution of the trauma was rapid and complete, often within a single session.

This discovery of an NLP system for dealing with trauma was, in effect, a rediscovery of Mesmer's 1780 techniques that had been used by Freud and hundreds of other psychotherapists up until the hypnosis scandals of the 1890s.

OTHER BILATERAL THERAPIES ENTER THE SCENE

In 1987, Francine Shapiro, then a graduate fellow in psychology at the University of California, was out for a walk one day when she noticed that side-to-side eye movements seemed to decrease the negative emotions connected with certain traumatic memories that she held. Shapiro carried this insight into her Ph.D. thesis in psychology, and from that developed what she called Eye Movement Desensitization, a technique by which she waved two fingers from side to side in front of a patient's eyes while having the patient call to mind a traumatic event. Her early experiences with this work convinced her that her technique could quickly heal trauma. She added to the practice a few classic psychotherapy techniques derived in part from Freud's talk therapy, and renamed the system Eye Movement Desensitization and Reprocessing (EMDR). Eye Movement Desensitization and Reprocessing has now been taught to tens of thousands of professionals and has been the subject of numerous studies that demonstrated its efficacy.[2]

Advocates of the system suggest that EMDR may be effective

because bilateral stimulation of the brain brings about some sort of neurological integration of emotional and intellectual processes involving the hippocampus, corpus callosum, and the two hemispheres of the brain. Others have suggested that EMDR's successes are simply a variation on Mesmer's original practice. While not using Mesmer's term *animal magnetism* or Braid's *hypnosis,* what has emerged in the past two decades since Shapiro first popularized EMDR are numerous similarly bilateral systems that purport to use left–right stimulation in various forms to heal trauma.

For example, Roger Callahan developed the systems called Thought Field Therapy (TFT) and the Callahan Techniques to help clients resolve trauma; he claims, not unlike Mesmer, that his system works because the "field" he works with is "an invisible structure in space that has an effect upon matter." His system involves the therapist tapping on classic acupuncture points along one side of the client's face, then on the opposite side of the client's torso, and then tapping on the client's wrist while the client watches the therapist move his or her hand in a large circle, then having the client alternately hum and count out loud (right-brain and left-brain functions).

In the late 1980s and early 1990s, Gary Craig developed a system called Emotional Freedom Technique (EFT) for treating trauma that draws on classic NLP systems of submodality shift, as well as on Freud's pre-1895 techniques of bilateral tapping on the face and body and back-and-forth eye movements. The EFT web site lists dozens of "cousins" of his energy-therapy system, with a wide variety of acronyms such as WHEE, TAT, NEAM, EDxTM, GTT, BSFF, WLH, MMT, and PET. What they have in common is that they all claim to heal trauma, using some form of bilateral stimulation of the eyes, ears, face, or body in the process.

All report success stories and claim to be able to easily prove their efficacy.

Another system that relies on bilateral movement and coordination is called Educational Kinesiology, or Brain Gym. Studies in Europe and the United States have shown that many of the Brain Gym exercises that use bilateral movement—rhythmic coordination of the right and left sides of the body—both help heal people of emotional disturbances and improve their memory, learning abilities, and general functioning.

As mentioned earlier, it's impossible to get upset while you're tossing a tennis ball from hand to hand. There is something very psychologically significant about bilateral movement.

BILATERAL EYE MOTION THERAPY IN ACTION

Stephen Larsen, Ph.D., is a longtime friend of mine and the biographer and former protégé of Joseph Campbell. Now retired from university teaching, Steven and his wife, Robin, run the Center for Symbolic Studies. As well, Stephen has a private psychology practice at the Stone Mountain Counseling Center in New Paltz, New York.

It was in this context that Stephen invited me to co-teach a weekend workshop with him at the Stone Mountain Counseling Center. His topic was broadly based in the ancient psychological, emotional, and spiritual healing systems of shamans, and mine was the modern systems designed to produce similar results through techniques such as NeuroLinguistic Programming.[3]

Our course, titled Hunters and Shamans, was designed principally for therapists, although every year that we presented it a few well-informed laypeople would show up. This particular year, one of them was a fellow whom I will call Ralph, a man who had been suffering for decades from severe post-traumatic stress disorder (PTSD).

Ralph was curious about what we had to say, and also hopeful that one of us would demonstrate the techniques we were discussing on him, and thus perhaps help his PTSD. Nothing else he had tried, from psychotherapy to drugs to biofeedback, had helped Ralph. Several times each day in the course of the preceding thirty years he would spontaneously and uncontrollably experience an eruption of panic, accompanied by an outburst of tears. These severe symptoms had rendered him unable to hold a job. He was distressed by his inability to earn a living and his need to survive on disability and Social Security payments.

Having told us all of this, Ralph said he had a past trauma that was troubling him and that he'd like to resolve. He said, further, that it was something he couldn't talk about without falling apart, so he was very interested to try something that didn't involve speaking the content of the event.

I explained that I was rostered as a psychotherapist in Vermont but not in New York, so anything I did would not be an attempt at therapy but would, instead, be a teaching demonstration for the purpose of showing Ralph and the others in the room the Eye Movement Therapy technique. Ralph came up to the front of the room and sat in the chair next to me that had been occupied by Stephen.

I told Ralph that, in the way this technique worked, the therapist would first ask the client where the client held the picture of her or his trauma. Ralph said that his memory picture was right in front of him, about two feet away, in a square area that roughly encompassed his chest. He began to tremble and tears came to his eyes as he pointed at the spot. I told Ralph and the group that it had been my experience that most people with PTSD held their traumatic memories in roughly the same place as Ralph did, and that when memories were located elsewhere, they were usually not the source of true PTSD symptoms. I then told Ralph that to do Eye Motion Therapy a therapist would *not* have the client look in the direction of the traumatic picture, but would instead direct her or his eyes everywhere else. As Ralph looked away from that spot, he regained his composure.

Ralph sat opposite me, facing me directly, our knees about six inches from one another's. I held a felt marker pen just above his eye level and told him that, with EMT, the therapist would ask the client to hold his head steady and just follow the tip of the pen with his eyes. I suggested that Ralph consider the intensity of the emotion he was experiencing right now as 100 on a scale of 0 to 100, and we'd check it again as we went along.

Then I began moving the pen around in regular, rhythmic patterns, from side to side across the top of his field of vision, going just to the edge of Ralph's field of vision, as if I was erasing a blackboard at that height. I continued this for about two minutes, then stopped.

"What's the intensity of the emotion now?" I asked.

Ralph glanced down and said, "Around eighty percent."

"Fine," I said, and repeated the process, this time moving through the center of his visual field as well as above it, but always being careful not to move the pen into the area where he said the painful picture was located. After another two or three minutes of having his eyes follow the pen from side to side, I stopped and asked how he was doing.

"It's down around sixty percent," he said.

We repeated the process again, and this time he said it went to about forty percent.

One of the keys to doing EMT and avoiding abreactions is not to enter the picture until the intensity is below 50 percent. When Ralph reported the emotional intensity to be at 40 percent, I again moved the pen from side to side but this time did it across his entire visual field, from top to bottom to top, as if I were thoroughly washing a blackboard. Whenever I noticed his eyes seize up for a moment and interrupt the smooth flow of motion as his eyes followed the pen, I'd revisit that area a few times until his eye motions were smooth at that spot.

After about two minutes of this, Ralph took a deep breath as his eyes were following the pen. Then he let the breath out, began to grin broadly, and chuckled under his breath.

I stopped the pen and asked, "What's up?"

He looked at me with an expression of mixed amusement and astonishment. "I can't believe what a dummy I've been all these years," he said.

"What do you mean?"

"I should have just let that go and gotten on with my life. Instead, I've wasted more than thirty years."

"Are we talking about the event that was bringing you to tears fifteen minutes ago?" I asked.

"We sure are," he said. "I was with a medivac unit in Vietnam, and after a really nasty firefight I called in two choppers to carry out the wounded. I was pretty sure all the enemy were dead, so after the choppers were loaded, I signaled them to take off. They got about two hundred feet up into the air when two rockets came out of the jungle and exploded both helicopters, raining parts and bodies on those of us on the ground." He shook his head with an expression of regret, although his tone was matter-of-fact. "I blamed myself for the deaths of those soldiers. Every day since that day in 1970 I've seen those choppers explode and heard those men screaming as they fell out of the sky."

"And now?"

He lifted his shoulders and dropped them. "I still remember it. But while you were doing that last pass there with the pen, suddenly it seemed like the pictures flattened out and took on the quality of an old newscast. And I heard my own voice in my head say, 'You did what you thought was right at the time. It was a mistake, but you did it with good intentions. You wanted to get those men to medical care, and you saved a lot of other lives while you were in that war. Now it's over and done with. There's nothing you can do about it, and it's time to forgive yourself and get on with your life. If nothing else, that's what the guys who died would want you to do, because it's what you would have wanted them to do if the situation had been reversed.' "

"And what's the intensity of the emotion right now?" I asked.

He shrugged again. "Close to zero. I mean, damn, it's been thirty years. It's over and done with."

It's been several years since Ralph participated in that teaching demonstration, and Stephen tells me that he's doing well in his life, has a job, and is no longer tortured by his past.

Battlefield trauma can be a shattering and life-altering event from which a person simply cannot recover. While eye-motion therapy and its variations—EMDR, TFT, and so forth—don't always work for severe trauma such as that experienced by many combat veterans, the frequent successes of EMT and its associated techniques demonstrate how powerful bilateral work can be at resolving past pains.

FIVE

Developing the Walking Your Blues Away Technique

The object of walking is to relax the mind. You should therefore not permit yourself even to think while you walk; but divert yourself by the objects surrounding you. Walking is the best possible exercise. Habituate yourself to walk very far."

THOMAS JEFFERSON

Seeing the correlations between bilateral therapies from the time of Mesmer to today, and knowing that bilateral eye motion in REM sleep is associated with healing traumas, I began to wonder: How would a person heal from trauma if there wasn't a mesmerist or energy therapist around and the trauma was too intense to be processed during REM sleep? How would humankind have handled trauma in an era without psychotherapists, hypnotists, and EMDR practitioners?

It was a sunny Vermont afternoon in the late spring of 2001 when I was first asking myself these questions. From my office window I could see some of the streets of Montpelier, and the people walking along those streets. I noticed that most people walked in a way referred to in Brain Gym as the "cross crawl"—the right arm swings forward with the forward swing of the left leg, then the left arm swings forward at the same time as the right leg. Back and forth, back and forth—right arm and left leg, left arm and right leg.

I realized with a start that this was bilateral, rhythmic motion! As people walk, they alternately engage the left and right hemispheres of the brain—the same aspects of the brain that the alternate-side eye movement and alternate-ear sound stimulation and alternate-side tapping therapies work to engage. *Could it be?* I wondered. Is it possible that the way our hunting/gathering ancestors relieved themselves of the burden of psychological trauma was by *walking back to the village from the hunt,* and that the walking itself stimulated the whole-brain psychological healing process?

Remembering that Francine Shapiro said she first discovered EMDR by having a difficult memory resolve itself while walking, I decided to try the same, but without moving my eyes from side to side.[1] I wanted to find out if the simple rhythmic bilateral activity of walking was enough to stimulate the brain to psychological healing.

The next morning I went for a walk from my home into downtown Montpelier and through some of the city's neighborhoods, a total of perhaps a half-hour's walk, a bit more than a mile. While walking rhythmically, using the cross crawl of a normal walker, I brought up a memory of a recent minor trauma—an embarrassing incident that occurred in a local drugstore. When I gave my name to the pharmacist, the woman standing next to me apparently recognized it and said, "Hi!" I wasn't sure if she was talking to me or to one of the people behind me, and so I was temporarily frozen in one of those social moments in which you are unsure of what to do. I meet many people, but rarely do I remember their names after just a first meeting. I'd recently given several speeches at local churches and done book signings. I'd been on local TV, and my radio show was broadcast on a local station, so it was possible that we had never actually met.

The pharmacist handed me my prescription and I left, never having responded to her. As I was leaving, however, I saw that she was staring at the floor, as if she was embarrassed. I left thinking that it must have been me she was speaking to, and that my shyness had caused her embarrassment. She was probably thinking I was some sort of insufferably arrogant snob, when in fact I was just caught in one of those socially awkward moments that you wish you could have left behind in high school.

For days afterward I tried to figure out who the woman was so that I could apologize, although my wife told me it was no big deal and that I should forget it. But to me it *was* a big deal—I thought about the experience daily. Every time I thought about it I relived the feeling of social anguish at not being able to acknowledge her, and the compounded and continuing embarrassment of thinking there was a person walking around town toward whom I'd behaved disrespectfully.

As I walked now, I mentally held the memory of that time in front of me, as though I was carrying a basketball in front of my chest. I walked normally through town, maintaining the rhythm of my walk but making no effort to move my eyes from side to side.

After about three blocks, I noticed that the colors in the

memory picture of the experience were beginning to blur and fade. And no matter how I tried to hold it in front of my chest, the location of the memory kept moving a few feet out and away from me, off to my left.

On the fourth block I suddenly heard my voice say silently to myself, "Hey, everybody's a little shy at heart, and most people would realize that you're not a snob but were just uncertain about how to react. And instead of thinking poorly of you, that woman is probably walking around feeling like an idiot because she spoke up and didn't get a reply. It would be nice if you could make it straight with her and both of you could feel better, but you don't have a clue who she is. So you may as well just let the whole thing go and resolve that the next time something similar happens, you'll answer the person even if it does feel awkward."

As my mind said this to me, the memory picture flattened out and lost most of its color. Suddenly I could see myself inside the picture instead of viewing the event from the outside. A feeling of relief washed over me, followed by a feeling of peace. I'd come to terms with the event and with myself.

This was not a form of self-therapy in which I engaged my cognition or familiar talk-therapy techniques. I hadn't set out to come up with a better story to tell myself about the event, or to alter my thinking about it. I was just carrying it with me as I walked, waiting to see if or how it would change. And change it did!

Later in the week I was talking with a client who is a psychologist. He felt "stuck" in a personal relationship that was very painful. He told me of all the past wounds around the relationship, and of how difficult he was finding it to separate himself from the other person, even though he knew that had to be done.

He'd come to an intellectual understanding of how toxic his

relationship was, but he hadn't been able to translate that into an emotional resolution. As a result, he spent hours every day obsessively thinking about this disintegrating relationship, to the point where it was interfering with virtually every other aspect of his life.

I told the client about my discovery of this simple Walking Your Blues Away system and suggested that he try it, asking him to report back to me how many minutes or miles it took him to resolve things, if that happened. He called me two days later to say it had taken him exactly seventeen minutes of steady walking, and that he could now pronounce himself "cured."

Emboldened by this success, I began recommending this system to all of my consulting clients. Because my practice is based almost entirely on doing short-term telephone consultations, mostly teaching NeuroLinguistic Programming techniques, with psychology-industry professionals such as psychiatrists, psychologists, psychotherapists, counselors, teachers, and coaches, I fortunately had a group of people who could easily understand the concept I was suggesting. And while my consulting is positioned as teaching and problem solving, at least half of the professionals who contact me for consultation are looking for techniques and ideas to resolve problems in their own lives as much as for their clients' lives and situations.

Every person I've shared this technique with, and who did it correctly (as opposed to listening to music while you walk or stopping to browse store windows, both of which interrupt the process), got resolution of his or her problem in less than a half hour. A few had to repeat the process for a few days in a row to wipe clear the final traces of emotional charge around an incident. It has not yet failed to work.

One of the mental health professionals who'd been in a class I taught on this technique about six months after 9/11 wrote to me about her personal use of it. Her husband travels frequently on business, and she'd been so severely traumatized by watching the video of the planes flying into the World Trade Center buildings over and over again that she was having regular nightmares and daily panic attacks whenever her husband was traveling by plane.

"I took the walk you suggested," she emailed me. "The walk *did* produce the hoped-for 'flattening' of the trauma of 9/11 and the resultant terror. Total time was about 20 minutes. I walked comfortably and observed nature around me, and drew in joy from the sights—and sounds—I encountered: a chipmunk staring back at me, the incredible call of an eagle overhead (I even spotted him!), the gentle 'moo' of the cows I passed."

She added that she'd still get anxiety "twinges" sometimes when Bush administration officials went on TV to talk about how "in danger" we all are. But she had anchored the "healing" experience of the walk with the music she played in her headset when she took the initial walk to deal with her daily anxiety attacks. The result was that, as she reported, "There have been tiny zaps of recurrence of the fear. When they pop up I hum the music, and the fear leaves. I believe that the recurrences have more to do with the fact that my husband is again traveling extensively than being spurred by the original trauma, and he and I are developing strategies to cope [with that separation anxiety]."

Upon further questioning, I learned that the fear this woman was describing around her husband's travels now have more to do with the normal and generalized concern for a loved one who is away—and the normal feelings of missing one's lover and friend.

They no longer were rooted in 9/11 anxiety at all. The walking experience had "healed" the 9/11 anxiety.

She added, "Thank you so very much for planting this [knowledge]! I'm now also using it in other such situations!"

Another professional in the mental health field for whom I'd done consulting work sent me a note that he was planning to try the Walking Your Blues Away technique after reading a rough first draft of this book.

"As you know," wrote Bob, "I have a big PTSD issue over the treatment I received from my uncle after my father died, and his cheating and stealing from the estate over a million dollars, which left me financially insecure."

He mentioned that he had done EMDR when his father died, and it helped him tremendously with the grieving process, "but the real trauma came when I couldn't stop, but only delay, my uncle from ripping me off!" His uncle had not only failed to notify Bob of the impending death of his father, but had actively been taking hundreds of thousands of dollars out of the family business as well.

"This has taken the life and energy out of me," Bob wrote. "While the anger rants walking around the house and most of the nightmares about it have decreased from several times a week to very occasional, I can get worked up about it in a few seconds if I think about it.

"I just don't have the energy or spirit to continue [living with] this level of PTSD. I'm literally worn out from worry and regrets about it. I'm hoping this walking process will help me to put the feelings that suck the life and energy out of me into the past, and allow me to go forward without the drain on my energy and motivation."

A week later Bob wrote to me again, after having tried the technique.

"I found that I was able to keep the issue floating in my head about 10 to 12 minutes of the entire walk to various degrees," he wrote. "I then 'felt' it under the surface as I looked at the new houses with for sale signs in front of them or people out in their yard in the evening. . . . Compared to what happened when I worked on this problem when I first became aware of it with EMDR in 1993, the difference was pronounced.

"Time is an element of this healing, and the issue is no longer current and ongoing, as it was just beginning then. But I definitely noticed a certain distance in feeling from the problem when I thought about it after the walk several hours later. I did not want to think about it any more, and it didn't seem important. I thought I'd get back to it Saturday, but didn't. . . . It really did reduce the energy around this issue. It now seems more a distant past memory than something currently simmering under the surface.

"The 'energy' for being upset about it is gone. For the first time I feel hope that I can finally get this behind me, and not let it influence my present. It will free me to go forward without carrying the weight of the past. That's how I feel now."

Noting that the walking technique had worked so well for him, a few weeks later Bob wrote that he was now looking forward to sharing it with his clients.

"My feeling is that I now have a tool I can use for myself and my clients," he wrote, "that can be used whenever that buzzing in the head starts about some hurt done to me (or them). Following the instructions to the best of my ability has brought great relief.

"Thank you for passing this on to me. I love the techniques I've learned from you and they always seem more direct and easy and avoid the formality of therapy sessions. They are the 'herb tea' of therapy: easily administered, and of immense value. I would choose this over traditional therapy in a second."

———∞∞∞———

SIX

How to Do a Walking Your Blues Away Session

All truly great thoughts are conceived while walking.

FRIEDRICH NIETZSCHE

There are five steps to correctly performing a Walking Your Blues Away session. They are:

- ▶ Define the issue.
- ▶ Bring up the story.
- ▶ Walk with the issue.
- ▶ Notice how the issue changes.
- ▶ Anchor the new state.

I will go into detail on each of the steps for you now.

DEFINE THE ISSUE

Before going for your walk, consider the issues that are still hanging around in your life that you feel are unresolved. This could range from past traumas, hurts, angers, or embarrassments to relationship issues with people you no longer have access to (including people who have died).

Don't worry that an issue might be too complex or something that happened over a long time. Many issues are multidimensional. What happens is that when the core issue is resolved, it rapidly begins the process of unwinding or "cleaning up" the peripheral associated issues.

Similarly, if you pick an issue that you may think is, itself, part of something larger, you'll notice after you've worked with it that the larger issue will also begin to resolve.

There's no specific right or wrong issue to work with. If you can think of it, visualize it, and get a feeling from it, then you can walk and work with it.

BRING UP THE STORY

Notice your story about the issue; *story* in this context refers to such thought patterns as "She was cruel toward me" and "He had no right to hurt me like that" and "Why did she have to die?" and "I'd like to get this job, but I don't know what to do to make it happen." There is always an internal story, with you and the object of the story at the center, and it's important to pull that story out so you can say and hear it explicitly. How would you describe the story—to yourself, in your most private and safe space—if you had to boil it down to a few words or a sentence or two? Once you have that, you have one of two tools to use in determining when your process has finished.

Another important tool is to notice the strength of the emotional charge associated with this event. Using a scale of 0 (truly don't care) to 100 (the most intense you have ever felt), come up with a number to rank the emotional charge connected with this event.

Not only will this number be useful in your work with the process; it will also be an excellent tool for gaining historical perspective, as often after a memory is resolved it's impossible to regain access to the original emotional charge (because it's been resolved). We can forget very quickly how important a past event once seemed.

WALK WITH THE ISSUE

Walking is pretty simple, but there are a few commonsense rules. Wear comfortable clothes and shoes. Don't bring along anything other than your ID, so you're not distracted by a hanging purse or a carried book: you want to be able to walk easily and to swing your arms comfortably.

Pick a route that is at least a mile long, and ideally two miles. At the average walking speed of three miles per hour, a mile is a twenty-minute walk. For those who walk fast comfortably, a mile takes approximately fifteen minutes.

Make sure the route matches your level of health: don't include hills or mountains if you have a heart condition and your doctor would warn you against overexertion. On the other hand, there's no need to exclude climbs that may get you out of breath if you're in good health and want to use your walk as aerobic exercise.

It's not necessary to pick a rural, suburban, or urban route. Anywhere you walk there will be things to distract you, from squirrels to the windows at Saks Fifth Avenue. The key is not in finding a distraction-free walking area—that's pretty much impossible. Rather, the key is to continue to remind yourself to hold your picture and/or feeling in front of you while walking.

Of course, nobody has perfect concentration. Most of us, in fact, are pretty attention compromised—after twenty or thirty seconds of walking we find our attention zooming off in some other direction. That's no problem—just keep reminding yourself to bring your attention back to the issue or goal, and again bring up the picture. The mind has a tremendous ability to pick up where it left off and continue processing things.

In reality, the total amount of "concentrated time" it takes your bilateral motion to resolve your issue or goal is probably just a matter of a few minutes—between five and ten minutes, in my experience. But to aggregate those few minutes, most people have to walk for a half hour or so, continuously reminding themselves to be present with the picture and feeling until all of the "remembering-to-do-it" moments add up to those five to ten total minutes.

One of the important keys to this process is to relax into it. It may take a few walks to get used to this manner of walking and not thinking—just like it took you a few tries to learn to ride a bicycle. To motivate yourself, though, think of the positive resolution that you're trying to achieve rather than engaging in any sort of internal dialogue that chastises you for past actions.

We're all wired to learn through trial and error. Learning how to quickly and easily do a Walk Your Blues Away session usually takes a few tries.

Remember: There is no failure. There is only feedback. Learn from the feedback and continue on.

NOTICE HOW THE ISSUE CHANGES

The submodalities—the primarily visual and auditory character-istics of a memory picture, such as how bright a memory picture is, where it's located, how clear it seems, whether it's in color or black-and-white, whether or not there's sound, whether it looks like a movie clip or a still picture, whether we see ourselves in the picture or see it as if we were watching from the outside—are the filing-system tags for the emotional brain. As the emotional value or the emotion attached to a picture/memory changes, the submo-dalities will change. When people walk with an unpleasant mem-ory, it's not uncommon for them to say that they see it beginning to disintegrate, or get dimmer, or lose its color, or move farther away (or even behind them). The dimming usually begins in a corner or in one part of the picture. As if it was an old photograph with a lit match held underneath it, part of the picture begins to distort and darken; then the change spreads across the entire picture, usually rather quickly.

Once this change has happened, people notice that the emo-tion they feel about the picture is now different. It's still possible to remember the event, but the feeling about the event is changed. Often the story of "I was hurt and it still hurts," for example, changes to something like, "I learned a good lesson from that, even if it was unpleasant." Present-tense pain becomes past-tense experience.

When you notice the picture changing (or the feeling changing, if that's all you could bring up), let the process proceed until you notice a perceptible shift in feeling and you no longer notice any changes taking place. Then ask yourself, "What's my story about this memory now?" If the process is complete, you'll discover that the story you're now telling yourself will be considerably healthier, more resilient, and more useful than the previous story. When the story changes to one that provides a positive frame, you're most likely finished with that memory for good.

ANCHOR THE NEW STATE

When the picture is well formed and you notice that your self-told story about the event has changed, anchor this new reality by reviewing it carefully—observe the way the picture has changed, listen to yourself repeat the new internal story, and notice the feelings associated with the new state. Notice all the ways it's changed. Think of other ways it may now be useful to you, even helpful. And, as you're walking back home or to your starting point, think about how you'd describe it if you were to choose to tell somebody else about it. (It's not at all necessary to tell anybody about it, but framing it in this way helps you clarify the new story.)

When you get home, consider writing something about your new experience, your new vision, your new story—an autobiographical narrative, like a diary entry, or something abstract, like a poem. If it's so personal and private that you don't want to write it down, just sit in a quiet and safe place and speak it out loud in private to yourself. These steps help anchor the new state, fixing it in its new place in your mind and heart, so it will be available to you as a resource—rather than a problem—in the future.

SEVEN

⠻

The Amnesia
of Healing

*I've learned that people will forget what you said,
people will forget what you did, but people will never
forget how you made them feel.*

MAYA ANGELOU

One of the most fascinating aspects of true psychological healing is how people who've been through a healing experience dismember, reassemble, and re-member their past. Psychological and emotional healing requires that the old stories of what happened to us, and that can fester inside, be examined, taken apart, and reassembled into a new whole that is supportive and healthy.

Because this is true healing, the result is a sort of amnesia about the original pain, not unlike the difficulty each of us has in remembering how much it hurt when we physically injured ourselves in the past.

In fact, one of the ways to know whether healing has occurred is to ask a person if they can remember clearly how much an original trauma hurt. They may say that they can, but the memory no longer brings tears to their eyes, no longer colors their view of the world, no longer nags at them daily. The amnesia isn't about details or facts—those remain intact. Rather, it is amnesia of *emotion*. A healed person has cut loose the old pain and let it drift away behind them into their past, where it's difficult to reach even should they want to reach it.

Ironically, this means that people, when healed, often don't realize the magnitude of the transformation that they themselves have experienced. Because in the present they can no longer re-experience the pain of that past, they have no clear basis for comparison between how they feel now and how they felt then. The result is that they'll often respond to questions about the healing—particularly more than a few weeks or months after the healing shift has occurred—with a shrug, as if to say, "Well, yeah, I feel fine now. But I wasn't so bad back then, was I?"

Of course, their friends and relatives remember well what a wounded wreck the person was. But the person has, as part of the healing process, disconnected so completely from the pain that it is no longer possible to remember it.

This is not an uncommon phenomenon: it happens in many other dimensions of emotional life. Ask a person about someone he or she was once in a relationship with, but is now completely out of the relationship and it's resolved and in their past. Odds are that person will have a very difficult time remembering what it was about the other person that attracted and held the two of them together. They may easily remember what they did together, but the feelings are no longer accessible.

This just makes psychological sense. If we didn't cut loose from old emotions as we move forward with life, they would constantly harass us. While joy states that derive from specific experiences are powerful tools we carry throughout our lives to help us confront daily dramas and traumas, past negative-emotional states that continue to visit us must be released for us to function in the now. In that "releasing" is also a "forgetting." Because the painful state is no longer available, people tend almost instantly to forget how much pain they were in—after all, the pain is no longer around for them to experience. They've let go of it.

This can be deflating news for therapists who employ bilateral systems, such as Walking Your Blues Away therapy, to bring about true, lasting healing. Your clients and friends don't remember how incapacitated they were, so they're not as amazed by the changes you've made happen as you are!

The good news here, though, is that when people have developed this sort of emotional amnesia about a past pain, they've really and truly been healed. Look for this as a landmark.

The other significant landmark that lets you know that healing has occurred—one that you'll often see on the very day, at the very moment that the big healing shift happens—is that the story the person tells about the past event changes. It usually shifts from some variation of "I was a victim of that" or "That really hurt me" to something like "I really learned from that" or "That wasn't such a big deal, and it's long over now."

PERSONALLY EXPERIENCING THE SHIFT

When you've been through this process yourself, you'll notice this shift, although it will be an intellectual realization rather than an emotional one.

Everyone, for example, has experienced a broken heart at one time or another in their lives. It's part of growing up, passing middle age, and growing old: it happens in every stage of life. Whether it's a teenage crush that devastates us when it doesn't work out or the loss of a friend or relative to disease or accidental death, we all get hurt. Ultimately, as Jim Morrison pointed out, "No one here gets out alive." Similarly, no one gets through life without being wounded.

Yet when you think back to some of the wounds you've experienced, odds are that most of them are now more intellectual than emotional memories. I still remember when my dearly beloved maternal grandmother died when I was a child: I was inconsolable. I remember myself sobbing, but I see it as a disconnected picture, in black-and-white tones, from a distant past. While I still miss her (and my paternal grandparents as well), the wound no longer rips me apart inside.

I still remember the first big love of my teenage years, and how she dumped me for a guy on the football team. I remember what I said and did, but I can't quite get a grasp on the frantic pain I know I experienced.

I still remember when my best friend from my high school years committed suicide. We had spent a summer living in tipis deep in the forest of northern Michigan on a spiritual quest when we were only seventeen. After high school he'd been drafted into the war in Vietnam. My friend came home from basic training for Christmas, put his revolver into his mouth, and pulled the trigger. I remember that event in my life, but I don't remember too. The excruciating pain is now gone, more than thirty years later—what is left is a memory that is wistful and sad but not agonizing.

None of these experiences was processed using any particular technique or therapy; they all resolved themselves, like skin heals over with a scab. No doubt there were processes I went through on the road to healing from these wounds—changing the stories I told myself, walking, discussing the events with others, and so on—but none was an "intentional" attempt to resolve trauma. I simply healed, as we all do from most of the vagaries and vicissitudes of life.

It's when we get stuck—unable to get past or around or through the "present-feeling" memory of a wound—that we need a technique such as Walking Your Blues Away or Thought Field Therapy or EMDR or NeuroLinguistic Programming to process, break loose from, and move out ahead of past traumas. Or when we simply want to speed up the normal healing and grieving processes we experience in life as the result of loss, disappointment, pain, or fear. We know we've been successful when the pain and trauma are only intellectual memories that can be handled once again without searing our flesh or blinding our vision.

EIGHT

Walking Your Blues Away with a Coach or Therapist

If I treat you as though you are what you are capable of
becoming, I help you become that.

JOHANN WOLFGANG VON GOETHE

Some people find themselves easily distracted when they walk, and they have a hard time—at least at first—doing Walking Your Blues Away therapy by themselves. Collaborating with some of the coaches and therapists I've trained over the years, I've developed a very simple protocol for the work. Therapists can take this as a rough outline. I present it in such a way that even nonprofessionals can do it with each other.

STEP 1: DEFINE THE ISSUE

The first step is to define where the person is stuck. What's the issue, the event, the problem, or the emotion that's hanging that person up?

Interestingly, it's *not* necessary for the therapist to know any details about the event or the trauma. People can keep their secrets. Because this work is done at the level of the *structure* of the *state*, it's not necessary to get caught up in the content of the memory or issue.

In fact, unless you're well trained in how to avoid getting stuck in the other person's dramas—their content—it's often most effective to do this exercise without ever asking or knowing what the details of the event/trauma/emotion are.

Working in the abstract like this accomplishes two things: It allows people to keep their secrets and privacy and it prevents an increase in the intensity of the emotions (a retraumatization) by engaging in discussion that repeatedly brings the issue or event back to consciousness. (These are the two main ways that "talk therapy" often wounds and re-wounds people.)

Thus, if you're dealing with content that you don't know the details of, it's useful to ask the walker to give the issue a name. It can be anything from a nonsense word ("Bzzlip!") to something meaningful to the walker but otherwise abstract ("Jessie," or "that time").

Once the event/trauma/emotion is defined, ask the walker to bring up a picture of the issue and to name where it exists in their kinesphere, the space around the body. If it's a true trauma, it will almost always be located directly in front of the chest. If it's something problematic but not traumatic, it may be located somewhere else relative to the body—behind, off to the side, or in the distance.

Ask the walker to point to the picture; if it's not directly in front of the chest, have the walker move it there for a moment. Ask the walker to determine, on a scale of 0 to 100, what the intensity of feeling was before placing the picture in front and then what the intensity was when the picture was placed in front of the chest. Note the shift in intensity when the memory picture is placed in front of the chest. Then have the person return the memory picture to where it was in the body's kinesphere initially. Rarely, moving the picture or feeling to a position in front of the person will produce an intense emotional reaction, such as bursting into tears. If this happens, tell the person to quickly return the picture to where it was initially, and then turn over the process to a trained professional.

Once you and the walker have identified the issue/event/feeling that will be the subject of your work together, it's time to head outside.

STEP 2: GO FOR A WALK

Choose a safe place to walk—"safe" in the sense that you're unlikely to run into people you know or be otherwise distracted by people or things you can't avoid. This doesn't rule out walking the streets of a city (even New York!)—you simply don't want to walk through a familiar neighborhood where you're likely to meet people you know, or through an area that is in some way associated with the trauma itself.

Define a route that will take at least twenty minutes, and then begin your walk. Take the first few minutes simply to relax, to notice your environment, to bring your attention and your client's thoughts to the present. To do this, suggest that the person walking with you notice what is to be seen in the immediate environment, then what can be heard, then what can be physically felt (the physical sensations of walking, the temperature, and so on). Ground yourselves in the present.

Make sure you're both walking in the natural cross-crawl fashion, with opposite arm and leg swinging forward with each stride, and that you are walking relaxed, with arms swinging naturally, not in an exaggerated way.

STEP 3: MAINTAIN DUAL AWARENESS OF PICTURE AND MOTION

When the walker is ready, suggest that he or she bring the image or feeling in front of the chest and hold the picture or emotion there as you walk. As you continue walking together, notice any changes in affect, body language, facial expression, breathing, or stride. If the walker breaks stride or changes the way he or she is walking, provide a gentle reminder to go back to a normal way of walking, while holding the picture at the same time.

Suggest that the walker notice how the body is being propelled forward first by the left foot, then by the right foot, then by the left again while the picture is being held in place in front of the body. The therapeutic effect is greatest when the walker is both conscious of the picture he or she is holding in front of the body and is conscious of the bilateral motion of the body, the shifting of weight and balance from right to left to right.

STEP 4: MAKE THERAPEUTIC SUGGESTIONS

One of the interesting aspects about suggestions made during this type of activity is how the unconscious mind of the other person handles them. In hypnosis it's nearly impossible to suggest that a person engage in an action that violates their basic code of behavior or isn't good or useful for them (or isn't at least neutral in that way). Similarly, the suggestions you make to the walker that may be less helpful or even counterproductive will generally be discarded, whereas the helpful ones will be used and processed.

Thus, as you're walking together, you may want to make occasional comments, in your own words, about how it's the natural course of living organisms to heal themselves, the way that when you scrape your knee it eventually scabs over and then finally the scab falls off and is left behind as new tissue and skin grows. Eventually there is no evidence—or only the smallest reminder—of the scrape in the first place.

Remind the walker to keep the picture in front of the chest, while simultaneously feeling the sensations of the bilateral motion of walking. Encourage the walker to notice that there is a left side and a right side to the field of vision, and even a left side and a right side to our auditory awareness.

You may want to remind the walker that it's the nature of life for every person to make mistakes, to have accidents happen, to cause and to be the recipient of problems, crises, and pain, and that the way we best recover from such experiences is to acknowledge them, apologize or forgive, let go, and move on with life, leaving the past to trail out behind us, where, forever over, it can never again harm us or others.

Remind the walker of the old saying "Nothing is true, but

thinking makes it so." The only way we can make sense of the world, the things that happen to us, and the constant stream of information that comes in through our senses is to tell ourselves stories about the things we see and experience. These stories help us make sense of life events, but sometimes these stories are either wrong or not useful and different stories are needed, and isn't it amazing how our unconscious mind can help us come up with new and more useful—and often even more accurate—stories about how things really are or once were?

You may want to note for the walker that it's perfectly normal—in fact, it's a good sign—if the picture of his or her past event is starting to change, becoming washed out or turning from color to black-and-white, or breaking up, or keeps trying to move behind the body (and into the past). When the walker is sure the picture, the memory story, is fully processed, he or she can feel free to let it change and move, as the unconscious mind best knows how to have it change and move to effect healing from that experience or trauma or pain or loss.

These kinds of suggestions, spoken somewhat rhythmically and as run-on sentences, tend to help the process along, while also sliding in beneath the radar of the walker's conscious mind. The use of classic "hypnotic language"—long statements that include lots of *ands* instead of periods or sentence ends—is a useful tool in helping people speed up their healing. On the other hand, if this is a manner of speaking that you haven't yet learned how to do in a way that sounds natural, just put the concepts into your own words.

None of this, of course, is necessary. Walking Your Blues Away therapy works when people do it alone. In fact, if you get over-involved in talking to the person with you, you may end up distracting the walker from holding the image and processing it as he or she walks. Try to achieve a balance of the occasional comment and a fair amount of silence. Being there and being supportive are enough. The main reason for going along with a person as he or she works through this process is simply to be a physical, present-moment reminder to hold the image before the body while walking and to stay grounded in the present moment as the experience of shifting the memory structure unfolds.

NINE

Walking for Creativity
and Problem Solving

The legs are the wheels of creativity.

Albert Einstein

Creativity and problem solving are psychologically similar processes. Both combine a linear approach—"How do I get from here to there?"—with the need to randomly access memories and ideas that may, in a linear world, seem completely unrelated.

One of the unique hallmarks of bilateral activity is that it gives access to the whole brain, making walking and other forms of bilateral work/play useful for enhancing creativity and problem solving. Resources and strengths, helpful learnings and experiences that date all the way back from childhood are available when walking, and can be brought to bear on current problems or creative endeavors.

Walking is a grounding experience, a step-by-step, moment-by-moment contact with the earth. Whether by some mystical force or some as yet unexplained psychological phenomenon, perhaps deeply rooted in our genes and stretching back over millions of years of evolutionary ancestry, feeling connected with the earth produces a liberating experience for most people.

Walking also provides us with a break from the state of normal everyday existence. Looking at the same walls, the same furniture, the same place and people often anchors us to a particular state of mind. When we go out for a walk, that state is broken, and new states of mind and emotion provoked by new sounds, sights, smells, and sensations offer access to new ways of knowing and understanding ourselves and our problems or opportunities.

The process for walking to solve problems or encourage creativity is straightforward. Decide on the issue you're going to bring to the walk, whether it's solving a business problem or figuring out how to finish a painting. Then, while walking, keep returning your mind to that specific issue, at the same time allowing it to freely roam in the intervals between your internal mental reminders. Letting your mind wander "randomly," yet at the same time "intentionally" bringing it back to the issue/problem at hand as often as you remember to, provides the space for both conscious and unconscious creative processes.

In his 1888 autobiography, *Ecce homo,* the famous German philosopher Friedrich Nietzsche tells the story of how the concept for his masterpiece *Thus Spoke Zarathustra* came as he was walking—something he did throughout his life when in need of inspiration. Nietzsche wrote down the core concept of the book during a walk in 1883, and added "6000 feet beyond man and time." A few weeks later he sat down and wrote the entire first part of the book in ten days.

In *Ecce homo* Nietzsche writes:

That day I was walking through the woods along the lake of Silvaplana; at a powerful pyramidal rock not far from Surlei I stopped. It was then that this idea came to me. . . .

Mornings I would walk in a southerly direction on the splendid road to Zoagli, going up past pines with a magnificent view of the sea; in the afternoon, whenever my health permitted it, I walked around the whole bay. It was on these two walks that the whole of Zarathustra One occurred to me, and especially Zarathustra himself as a type; rather he overtook me.

Describing how walking would activate his creative processes and cause concepts to fall into consciousness fully formed, Nietzsche added: "One hears, one does not seek; one accepts, one does not ask who gives; like lightning, a thought flashes up, with necessity, without hesitation regarding its form—I never had any choice."

Another quick technique that can aid in both problem solving and enhancing creativity is to ask the creative part of you to participate in the walk. This is essentially what Nietzsche did—whenever he walked he fully expected the creative part of his mind to make an appearance. Although this may sound a bit odd, try this simple exercise right now and you'll discover how real and useful it can be.

After you finish reading this paragraph, put the book down, close your eyes, and ask yourself, "Is there a creative part of me in here?" Do it now.

Nearly everybody will hear or sense some sort of a "Yes" answer to that question, because we are complex beings with different internal mental and emotional aspects of ourselves that have taken responsibility for different tasks in our lives.

When you're going to walk for problem solving or for encouraging creativity, before you go on the walk ask the creative part of you if it will participate in the process by tossing out possibilities and helping you see or hear or get new ideas as you're walking. You may also want to ask if there's a part inside you that has taken responsibility for the creative project or problem you're trying to solve. When that part of you agrees, ask it if it is willing to receive some help from your creative self. Again, the answer is almost always, "Yes!"

Once you've accessed both of those parts of yourself and put them in touch with one another, go for the walk.

TEN

Walking to Create a
Motivational State

*People often say that motivation doesn't last. Well, neither
does bathing—that's why we recommend it daily.*

ZIG ZIGLAR

In his 1937 classic *Think and Grow Rich,* Napoleon Hill shared
the secret that steel baron Andrew Carnegie used to transform
himself from a penniless Scottish immigrant into one of the richest
men in America. That secret, Hill reveals, is to bind a clear vision
of a future you want (in the case of his book, a future filled with
riches) with a strong and positive emotional state.

Hill wasn't the first to observe how motivational states work.
Three centuries before Christ was born, Plato wrote *Protagoras,*
a story of a discussion between the sophist Protagoras and Plato's
teacher, Socrates. In this classic example of Socratic dialogue, the
two men struggle with questions such as "Why do the sons of

good fathers often turn out ill [or good]?" and "Surely knowledge is the food of the soul?"

Socrates speaks directly to motivation and results, asking Protagoras, "And what is done strongly is done by strength, and what is weakly done, by weakness?" Plato tell us: "He [Protagoras] assented."

Following a lengthy discussion of how people are raised and what they learn, one of the conclusions the men come to is that people are more strongly motivated by what they consider close than by what they consider far away, be it in distance or in time.

Or, as King Solomon is purported to have said a thousand years earlier, "When desire cometh, it is a tree of life" (Proverbs 13:12).

We are all, always, choosing between moving toward pleasure and moving away from pain. Every single minute is filled with one or the other: we're never neutral.

Moving away from pain is the "hotter" of these two, but strategies that move us toward pleasure provide long-term, compelling, inexorable motivation. A good analogy is that moving-away-from-pain strategies are like lightning, producing rapid but short-lasting (and sometimes painful) jerks away from what we fear, whereas moving-toward-pleasure strategies are like gravity—inexorable, continuous, and ultimately a means for bringing us to our goals.

The key to making powerful moving-toward-pleasure choices and connecting them to our goals is anchoring a positive vision of the future we want with a powerful positive emotional state. Motivational teachers over the years have proposed many fine techniques to accomplish this—putting up note cards with motivational slogans on mirrors and refrigerators, reading a motivational statement every morning and evening, listening to tapes of motivational speakers regularly—but all eventually bring us to the same place: creating a powerful vision of the future that is bright, shining, and desirable.

Using the Walking Your Blues Away technique, you can build and anchor strong positive motivational states. The process is quite straightforward:

- ► While walking, visualize possible future states.
- ► Select the one that seems optimal and that you want to focus on.
- ► While you're walking, hold the visualization in front of you, at whatever distance or location seems most comfortable and appropriate.
- ► While walking and holding this future ideal, remember times in the past when you were able to accomplish similar things or had great successes or desires fulfilled.
- ► Allow the emotional state of the positive memories to fill and suffuse the hoped-for future state.
- ► See yourself in the picture clearly—how you're dressed, what you're doing, how you're standing.
- ► When the positive future state is clear and makes you smile, stand up a bit straighter and feel powerfully good. Create a word, sound, gesture, or posture to anchor the state.
- ► Repeat the anchoring reminder a few times until it once again brings up the feeling of success in your body, then finish your walk.

Having done this, you can then put up reminders around the house—the cards on the refrigerator and mirrors with a word or two that remind you of your future goals. Whenever you see these, you then assume the posture and make the sound or gesture that re-accesses that state, remembering your goals and letting the full positive intensity of the enthusiastic emotion fill you.

Over time—often over a surprisingly short time—you'll discover that you are achieving your goals. Programming your unconscious mind like this, you'll begin to see opportunities and chances where before you would have missed or ignored them. You'll find yourself moving toward your positive future as if it were drawing you in the same inexorable straight line that drew Newton's apple from the tree.

ELEVEN

Walking to Improve Physical Health

Walking is man's best medicine.

HIPPOCRATES

Walking may well be the best single exercise there is for human beings. We're designed to walk. Through most of our history, we walked several miles a day in search of food, water, and firewood—as indigenous people do to this very day.

Unlike running, walking rarely causes injuries. It is infinitely variable—you can walk fast or slow; uphill, downhill, or straightaway; you can carry small weights in your hands or strapped to your ankles to increase the cardiovascular effect; or you can simply walk comfortably and freely.

Not only are our bodies designed to be able to walk, they *require* walking to work right.

Walking exercises the heart and lungs and stimulates the

pumping of the lymphatic system. There are more than six hundred lymph nodes in the body; they are an essential element of our immune system. But unlike the circulatory system, which has a heart to push blood through our veins and arteries, the lymph system relies on gravity. Every time you take a step, your entire lymph system is stimulated and the flow of lymphatic fluids increases.

Hundreds of studies have found that people who walk for at least fifteen to thirty minutes a day are healthier than people who don't. They contract fewer diseases, are less likely to get cancer, have lower risks of heart attack and stroke, and have better bone density.

Walking improves digestion and decreases the risk of intestinal cancers, validating the old Chinese proverb that suggests a person take a walk after eating a meal, counting one step for each time you chewed during the meal. Regular walking reduces the risk of type II diabetes and reduces the insulin dependency of people who have already developed that disease. It recalibrates the body's energy and energy-storage (fat) systems, so the body becomes trimmer and more efficient.

Walking helps the kidneys stay clean and clear; like the lymphatic system, the kidneys rely to some extent on gravity. Walking helps maintain your joints by flexing them and increasing the production of joint-lubricating fluids. In this regard, some researchers suggest that walking helps diminish, or at least ward off, some types of arthritis.

Regularly walking fast enough, far enough, or uphill enough to elevate your heart rate even a small amount will cause your arteries, veins, capillaries, and heart to recalibrate toward greater efficiency. Over time, this leads to a decreased resting heart rate and a dramatic reduction in the chances of developing cardiovascular diseases throughout your life.

Numerous studies have associated walking with a reduction of depression, anxiety, and sadness, even in parts of the world that have long and dark winters. Although most assume this is because walking increases blood flow—and, thus, the flow of oxygen and nutrients to the brain—it may also be because of the fact that walking is a bilateral motion.

For example, a study done in 1999 at Duke University found that a brisk thirty-minute walk three times a week was more effective in relieving patients of symptoms of depression than either the drug Zoloft *or* the drug plus the exercise. A follow-up study found the exercise-only patients were also less likely to have a recurrence of their depression. As Duke University noted in 2000:

> After demonstrating that 30 minutes of brisk exercise three times a week is just as effective as drug therapy in relieving the symptoms of major depression in the short term, Duke University Medical Center researchers now have shown that continued exercise greatly reduces the chances of the depression returning.

Last year, the Duke researchers reported on their study of 156 older patients diagnosed with major depression, which, to their surprise, found that after sixteen weeks, patients who exercised showed statistically significant and comparable improvement relative to those who took antidepression medication and those who took the medication and exercised.

> The new study, which followed the same participants for an additional six months, found that patients who continued to

exercise after completing the initial trial were much less likely to see their depression return than the other patients. Only 8 percent of patients in the exercise group had their depression return, while 38 percent of the drug-only group and 31 percent of the exercise-plus-drug group relapsed.[1]

The Duke researchers were particularly startled when they found that people who exercised just as much as the exercise-only group but also took the antidepressant drug had a much harder time shaking their depression. "Researchers were surprised," said the Duke University press release, "that the group of patients who took the medication and exercised did not respond as well as those who only exercised."

While nobody is sure why taking an antidepressant pill with exercise would dramatically reduce the effectiveness of exercise to relieve depression (and the pill wasn't as effective, either), one possibility is that when a person is on an antidepressant medication, they're less likely to be thinking of the issues at the core of their depression. (This is one of the things that antidepressant drugs do, after all—they "push away" painful thoughts.) Therefore, when the bilateral exercise was engaged in by the exercise-and-drug group, they didn't mentally or emotionally have the "issues in need of processing" easily "available" to be chewed up and digested by the bilaterality of the exercise.

There is virtually no downside to walking, as long as your doctor says you're in a condition that allows for it. And to gain these benefits, walking need not be strenuous or time consuming. Walking an approximate mile—fifteen minutes a day—just three to five times a week produces measurable improvements in nearly all the indices previously mentioned.

Depending on whether you walk in the country, the suburbs, or the city, walking also reconnects us with the natural world and with our fellow human beings. Regularly walking with your spouse, children, or a close friend is a great way to maintain connections and to spend some time together.

There's even evidence that conditions such as attention deficit hyperactive disorder (ADHD) benefit from walking—or at least from spending time outdoors, which virtually requires walking, as opposed to indoor activities such as basketball and weightlifting. In a study published in the September 2004 issue of the *American Journal of Public Health*, the authors noted that for children diagnosed with ADHD, being outside part of every day significantly reduced the symptoms of ADHD. As the study's abstract said: "In this national nonprobability sample, green outdoor activities reduced symptoms [of ADHD] significantly more than did activities conducted in other settings, even when activities were matched across settings. Findings were consistent across age, gender, and income groups; community types; geographic regions; and diagnoses."[2]

Fish swim, birds fly, humans walk. Start walking today!

Share It with Others (The Best Things in Life Are Free)

Thousands of candles can be lighted from a single candle,
and the life of the candle will not be shortened. Happiness
never decreases by being shared.

BUDDHA

When Franz Anton Mesmer discovered bilaterality, he succeeded in turning it into a source of fame and cash for himself. Even as his system became increasingly controversial in Europe, Mesmer was suggesting that only people trained by him in how to bring down "animal magnetism" from the skies should be authorized to perform his early form of bilateral therapy.

In many ways, the history of psychology and psychiatry (and religion) has been the history of people attempting to hold on to power and generate wealth by making their knowledge available exclusively through their own institutions.

But if it's true—as I'm certain it is—that we're designed to be as psychologically self-healing as we are physically self-healing, and that walking is a key part of that process, then it seems important to put this information out into the public domain and let people share it widely. After all, this isn't psychology or psychiatry or any sort of medicine: it's simply a return to the way our body and mind were designed to self-heal.

When you've had the experience of this technique working for you, share it with a friend! Step by step (consider where that metaphor may have come from!) we will heal ourselves, our friends and family, and, ultimately, the planet.

Notes

⊶⊷

INTRODUCTION

1. From the American Psychiatric Association at www.psych.org.
2. Lori Lebovich, "No Sex Please: We're Medicated," published online at Salon.com, July 1997.
3. E. E. Werner and R. S. Smith, *Vulnerable but Invincible: A Longitudinal Study of Resilient Children and Youth* (New York: McGraw-Hill, 1982).

CHAPTER 1

1. Anahad O'Connor, "The Reach of War: The Soldiers; 1 in 6 Iraq Veterans Is Found to Have Stress-Related Disorder," *New York Times*, July 1, 2004.
2. As clinical psychologist Mark Grant notes about the bilateral therapy Eye Motion Desensitization and Reintegration (EMDR) at www.overcomingpain.com/spec.html: "Trauma victims, who were treated with EMDR and given a SPECT brain scan, pre and post EMDR, showed reduction in some of the neurological abnormalities associated with their condition" (van der Kolk, 1996). "Specifically, the anterior cortex of the cingulate gyrus was activated. . . . And there was a lateralization effect as a result of the left hemisphere (Broca's area) becoming reactivated" (van der Kolk, 1996).

   "Nicosia (1994) found that examination of EMDR clients by electroencephalography (QEEG) revealed a normalization in the slower brain wave activity of the two cortical hemispheres. . . .

"This tentative evidence that EMDR works to correct neurological abnormalities underlying trauma, which have parallels with pain, suggests that it might also be efficacious with pain."

CHAPTER 2

1. James Wyckoff, *Franz Anton Mesmer: Between God and Devil* (New York: Prentice Hall, 1975).
2. Ibid.
3. Ibid.
4. James Braid, *Magic, Witchcraft, Animal Magnetism, Hypnotism, and Electrobiology* (London: John Churchill, 1841).
5. James Braid, M.D., "Hypnotism or Neurypnology, the Rationale of Nervous Sleep," *Medical Times,* 1842, and "Electro-Biological Phenomena and the Physiology of Fascination," *Medical Times,* 1855. Both reprinted with a foreword by Arthur Edward Waite in London in 1899. Compiled and republished with a new foreword by J. H. Conn, M.D., in 1960 (New York: Julian Press).
6. Sigmund Freud and Josef Breuer, *Studies on Hysteria* (New York: Basic Books, 1957).
7. *Hypnose,* by Sigmund Freud, first published in German in Anton Bum's *Therapeutisches Lexikon* in 1891, reprinted in English in *Foundations of Hypnosis: From Mesmer to Freud* by Maurice M. Tinterow, M.D. (Springfield, IL: Charles Thomas, publisher, 1970).
8. Freud and Breuer, *Studies on Hysteria.*
9. Josef Breuer and Sigmund Freud, *On the Psychical Mechanism of Hysterical Phenomena: Preliminary Communication* (1883).
10. Ibid.
11. Ibid.
12. Ibid.
13. Ibid.
14. George Du Maurier, *Trilby,* originally published in 1894 (New York: Kessinger, 2004).
15. Ibid.
16. www.druglibrary.org/schaffer/cocaine/freud.htm.
17. G. Lebzeltern, "Sigmund Freud und Cocaine," *Wien Klin Wochenschr* 95 (21) (November 1983).

18. Translated by A. A. Brill in the Encyclopedia Britannica, cited in *Basic Writings of Sigmund Freud* (New York: Random House, 1983).

CHAPTER 3

1. Thomas Jefferson, *Notes on Virginia, 1784–85.*
2. Charles Darwin, *Descent of Man.* First published in London, 1871.
3. Daniel Quinn, *Ishmael* and *My Ishmael* (New York: Bantam Books, 1995 and 1998).
4. Walter J. Ong, *Orality and Literacy* (Oxford: Routledge, 1982).
5. Leonard Shlain, *The Alphabet Versus the Goddess: The Conflict Between Word and Image* (New York: Penguin, 1999).
6. Peter Farb, *Man's Rise to Civilization, as Shown by the Indians of North America from Primeval Times to the Coming of the Industrial State* (New York: Avon Books, 1976).

CHAPTER 4

1. Wikipedia.
2. The web site www.emdr.org has many of these studies available.
3. I am certified and licensed by the Society of NeuroLinguistic Programming as both an NLP practitioner and an NLP trainer. I learned much of what I know on the topic from Richard Bandler.

CHAPTER 5

1. Francine Shapiro tells this story in her book *Eye Movement Desensitization and Reprocessing* (New York: Guilford Publications, 1995).

CHAPTER 11

1. From the Duke University Medical Center News Office web site: www.dukemednews.org/news/article.php?id=119.
2. Frances E. Kuo, Ph.D., and Andrea Faber Taylor, Ph.D., "A Potential Natural Treatment for Attention-Deficit/Hyperactivity Disorder: Evidence from a National Study," *American Journal of Public Health* 94: 1580–1586.

Index